An Introduction to
THERAPEUTICS FOR CHIROPODISTS

An Introduction to
Therapeutics for Chiropodists

PETER J. READ
F.Ch.S., Dip.F.E.

FORMER HEAD OF THE
CHELSEA SCHOOL OF CHIROPODY

THE ACTINIC PRESS

This second edition (reprint revised) published in 1978
by Actinic Press
A division of Cressrelles Publishing Company Limited
10 Station Road Industrial Estate, Colwall,
Malvern, Worcestershire WR13 6RN

Reprinted 1979, 1984, 1985, 1990, 1994, 1996

First published by Bailliere Tindal and Cox in 1957
Second edition published by Actinic Press in 1972

ISBN: 0 900024 17 8

Printed and bound in Great Britain by
BPC (Wheatons) Limited

TABLE OF CONTENTS

EDITOR'S PREFACE TO THE
SECOND EDITION (REPRINT)

IN reprinting the second edition of *Therapeutics for Chiropodists* the opportunity has been taken for making a number of important amendments. These have been fitted in to the text where appropriate and because of the need to retain the original pagination there may be some awkwardness of style in certain passages. The addendum to the index will indicate where new material has been added.

I am once again greatly indebted to members of the staff of the Chelsea School of Chiropody particularly to Mr. D. Ashcroft, Mr. B. Berry, Mr. M. Hobday and Mr. C. Shipman for their help in producing this reprint.

Peter J. Read

London
September 1977

EDITOR'S PREFACE TO THE SECOND EDITION

IN presenting the second edition of *Therapeutics for Chiropodists* I am grateful for the encouragement of colleagues throughout the profession. With the accent on team teaching I have enlisted the help of many of the staff at the Chelsea School of Chiropody in revising various sections and I pay tribute to their enthusiasm and support. At the same time I accept responsibility both for the format and content of the book as a whole and for any errors of commission or omission.

Those who have helped in the production of the new edition include Mr. T. T. Coates and Mr. J. Foulston who have also helped with much of the editorial and administrative work and also Mr. I. S. C. Anderson, Mr. D. Ashcroft, Miss R. Avery, Mrs. C. Martin, Mr. M. Hobday, Mrs. H. Lilley, Mr. W. M. Long, Mr. J. Sanders, Mrs. J. Shanks, Mr. A. W. Swallow, Mr. B. Taylor, Mr. J. W. J. Turvey and Mr. R. Winder.

One of the two great problems has been to decide on which treatments to include and which to omit. Many of the older treatments have still been included even where they are old-fashioned by modern standards. I hope, however, that this book will help to give older chiropodists who have been in practice for many years an insight into modern drugs and methods of treatment. The second great problem is one of standard. The pharmacology of many drugs is extremely complex and it is tempting to dwell on abstruse and difficult points. I have tried to produce a work of sound scholarship with a bias towards practical applications at the same time as giving a clear, if simplified, theoretical basis for the rationale of chiropodial therapeutics.

Peter J. Read

London
July, 1971

AUTHOR'S PREFACE TO THE FIRST EDITION

THE object of this book is twofold: first, to give information of practical value concerning the drugs used in chiropody and, second, to give a theoretical background to the treatment of various conditions. I have allowed myself a wide degree of latitude in discussing the treatment of various conditions since, in order to understand treatment, normal physiology and pathology must first be understood. For this reason inflammation in its various aspects is discussed at length, together with the healing processes and the body's reaction to infection. The fact that the pathology in certain sections, as for instance that on corns and callus, can be a matter only of hypothesis should constitute a challenge to others as well as to myself. In addition to giving details of specific treatments, I have endeavoured, wherever possible, to formulate general principles upon which treatment may be based. I hope that the approach to therapeutics based upon physiological and pathological considerations may lead to the development of new treatments.

Throughout the book I have adopted the nomenclature of the British Pharmacopœia and the British Pharmaceutical Codex, using the English titles which are now the official first titles; in the monographs the Latin titles are given in parenthesis. The use of quotation marks indicates a proprietary preparation and of capital letters that the item referred to is the official preparation.

It is not possible for me to acknowledge the sources of the various treatments I have described, nor do I make any claim to originality but I have incorporated many helpful suggestions and ideas from others, for which I am most grateful. In particular, I extend my warmest thanks to my colleagues in the Department of Chiropody, Chelsea Polytechnic, for their help and advice. This book, therefore, presents a body of information drawn from many sources and assembled in a form in which it is hoped will prove of practical value to both students and practitioners.

Peter J. Read

London
October, 1956

PART ONE

CHAPTER I

TYPES OF PREPARATION

SELECTION of the type of preparation in which a drug is used depends on the possible methods of dispensing the medicament concerned and on the practitioner, who selects the preparation best suited to the needs of the patient. For example, aminacrine hydrochloride, one of the acridine group of antiseptics, has been dispensed as:

   (i) A solution in water, or in normal saline.
  (ii) A buffered solution.[1]
 (iii) A solution in ethyl alcohol or in iso-propyl alcohol.
  (iv) A cream (emulsion).[2]
   (v) An ointment.
  (vi) A jelly.
 (vii) A gelatin paste.
(viii) An impregnated gauze.

In this example, while the efficiency of the drug, aminacrine hydrochloride, may vary with the different vehicles used, its essential property, that of being antiseptic, does not vary. The choice made by the chiropodist will depend on the incidental properties of the base and will be governed by such factors as the condition of the patient's skin, the type of dressing to be used, the site of the application, etc. In contrast, to take the example of iodine, when this is dispensed as a solution its bactericidal and fungicidal properties predominate, but in ointment form it is employed chiefly as a rubefacient. Phenol, which has antiseptic properties when dispensed in aqueous solutions, has little or no germicidal or antiseptic properties when prepared in alcohol, in oil or in purely fatty bases. It is very important that the chiropodist should know the various types of preparations which are available and the general properties of each group.

The preparations used in chiropody may be divided up in several ways. They may be liquid, semi-solid or solid, or they may be solutions, suspensions or mixtures; or they may be subdivisions of these groups. In any case the grouping is quite arbitrary, and this is reflected in the official pharmaceutical names of the various preparations. These titles were formerly given in Latin but in 1953 they were changed to English.

In the list below, the Latin name is given in parenthesis.

1. Preparations which take their pharmaceutical title from the type of base in which they are prepared

(a) *Collodions* (Collodi-um, pl. -a) are preparations of drugs in a Collodion base, e.g. Salicyclic Acid Collodion B.P.C.

(b) *Ointments* (Unguent-um, pl. -a) are semi-solid preparations in various fats, oils and waxes. These are discussed more fully below.

(c) *Pastes* (Past-a, pl. -ae) are preparations containing a high proportion of a powder mixed with soft paraffin or with liquid paraffin or in a non-greasy base.

(d) *Plasters* (Emplastr-um, pl. -a) are plastic or resinous masses which are spread on some supporting material, e.g. Zinc Oxide Self-adhesive Plaster B.P.C.

(e) *Solutions* (Liquor, pl. -es) are solutions of drugs in water or alcohol, e.g. Ferric Chloride Solution B.P.C. (aqueous), Weak Iodine Solution B.P. (spiritous).

(f) *Tinctures* (Tinctura, pl. -ae) are preparations of drugs of *Vegetable Origin* in alcohol, e.g. Benzoin Tincture B.P.C.

2. Preparations which take their pharmaceutical title from the way in which they are applied

(h) *Liniments* (Liniment-um, pl. -a) are liquid or semi-liquid preparations intended for external use only, where the skin is unbroken. Soothing liniments, e.g. Calamine Liniment B.P., 1948, may be applied on cotton dressings or may be painted on. Stimulating liniments, e.g. Methyl Salicylate Liniment B.P.C., are applied with friction.

(i) *Lotions* (Loti-o, pl. -ones) are dabbed or painted on to the skin or are applied as wet dressings to the skin. They may be solutions in water or alcohol, e.g. Lead Lotion B.P.C., or they may be suspensions in water, e.g. Calamine Lotion B.P.

(j) *Paints* (Pigment-um, pl. -a) are preparations intended for application to the skin or a mucous surface, e.g. Magenta Paint B.P.C., Castellani's Paint.

3. Preparations which take their pharmaceutical title from the use to which they are put

(k) *Creams* (Crem-or, pl. -ores) are emulsions which are intended for external use only, e.g. Proflavine Cream B.P.C., c.f. *Emulsions* which are intended for internal use.

(*l*) *Dusting-powders* (Conspers-us, pl. -i) are powders intended for external use only, e.g. Chlorhexidine Dusting Powder B.P.C., c.f. *Powders* which are intended for internal use.

It will be noticed that in many cases a preparation could be placed in more than one of the above groupings. Crystal Violet and Brilliant Green Paint B.P.C. might easily be grouped with the Solutions since it is a solution of brilliant green and crystal violet in water and alcohol; Compound Benzoin Tincture B.P. might be grouped with the Paints, etc.

To avoid confusion, wherever Emulsion, Paint and Cream are used with a capital letter they must be taken in the specific pharmaceutical sense, whereas, when they are spelt with a small letter they are to be taken in a general sense.

Many of the pharmaceutical preparations which the chiropodist encounters are solutions, generally of solids in liquids. A solution may be defined as a homogeneous molecular mixture; that is to say that the molecules of the dissolved substance, the solute, are dispersed evenly throughout the molecules of the solvent which is the component having the same physical state as the solution itself. In the case of a solution of salt in water, the water is in the same physical state as the salt-solution and therefore the water is the solvent and the salt is the solute.

A given solvent will dissolve only so much of a given solute. The amount of substance which will dissolve depends on the solute, the solvent and the temperature of the solvent. Thus at 20° C., 1 part of sodium chloride will dissolve completely in 3 parts of water or 10 parts of glycerin. At the same temperature 1 part of boric acid is soluble in 20 parts of water or in 4 parts of glycerin. It is not possible to produce an aqueous solution of boric acid stronger than 5 per cent. If more than 1 part of boric acid is mixed with 20 parts of water, then not all the boric acid will dissolve and there will be a white sediment in the solution. Such a solution is said to be "saturated", and it is a general rule that no solution is regarded as being saturated unless there is some undissolved solute in the solvent. Generally an increase in temperature means that more of a substance will dissolve in a given quantity of solvent.

Pharmaceutical percentages are conventional, the term "per cent" is used according to circumstances with one of four meanings.

Per cent w/w (weight in weight) expresses the number of grammes of active substance in 100 g. of product.

Per cent v/v (volume in volume) expresses the number of millilitres of active substance in 100 ml. of product.

Per cent w/v (weight in volume) expresses the number of grammes of active substance in 100 ml. of product.

Per cent v/w (volume in weight) expresses the number of millilitres of active substance per 100 g. of product.

Solutions of liquids are expressed as percentage volume in volume; solutions of solids in liquids as percentage weight in volume, and solutions of gases in liquids as percentage weight in weight.

This convention explains the apparent anomaly of a 200 per cent Silver Nitrate Solution. Silver nitrate is extremely soluble in water and 100 ml. of water will dissolve 200 g. of silver nitrate. Thus 100 ml. of saturated solution of silver nitrate in water will contain 200 g. of silver nitrate hence it is a 200 per cent solution in pharmaceutical terms.

When a substance is not soluble in the vehicle in which it is dispensed, it may be prepared in a variety of ways. Those commonly encountered are the *mixture*, as in the case of foot powders where the solid constituents are merely mixed together; the *suspension*, where the insoluble medicament, usually a solid, is evenly dispersed throughout a vehicle which is usually liquid or semi-liquid in nature; and the *emulsion*. An emulsion consists of two mutually immiscible parts or phases and generally one phase is aqueous (watery) and the other phase is oily in nature. It is well known that oil and water will not mix and that if they are shaken up together, although coarse globules of oil may be dispersed temporarily throughout the water, or vice versa, the two phases will soon separate again. If an agent such as soap is added to the water, it is possible to disperse the oil evenly throughout the water in small globules and for the oil to re-

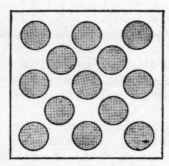
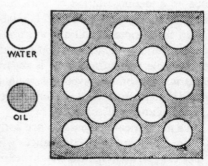

Oil-in-water emulsion
Disperse Phase—oil;
Continuous Phase—water

Water-in-oil emulsion
Disperse Phase—water;
Continuous Phase—oil

FIG. 1

main so dispersed. This dispersion of the oil in the water is called an *emulsion* and the soap an *emulsifying agent* or *emulgent*. If small globules of the oily phase are dispersed throughout the watery phase it is known as an oil-in-water emulsion and the oil is said to be in the disperse phase and the water in the continuous phase. If small globules of the watery phase are dispersed throughout the oily phase it becomes a water-in-oil emulsion with the water in the *disperse phase* and the oil in the *continuous phase*. (Fig. 1.)

The molecules of an emulsifying agent have the property of being partly soluble in water (hydrophilic, or water-loving) and partly soluble in oil or fat (lipophilic, or fat-loving). The ideal situation for such a molecule is to have its hydrophilic end in water and its lipophilic end in oil. Fig. 2 shows a vessel containing separate layers of oil and water. Here the area of oil in contact with water, the interface, is at its minimum, but in Fig. 3 where the oil has been split

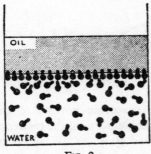

FIG. 2

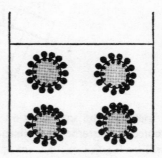

FIG. 3

up into globules the area of the oil-water interface has been increased. When the emulgent is introduced into the oil and water before the two are shaken up there is not enough room for all the molecules of the emulgent to have, as it were, their heads in water and their tails in oil, because the area of the oil-water interface is insufficient. (Fig. 2.) When the oil is split up into globules the area of the interface is increased so that there is sufficient room for all the molecules to occupy their ideal situation. (Fig. 3.)

The molecules of the emulgent, besides being partly fat-, and partly water-soluble, are also asymmetrical with regard to shape. In some molecules, for example those of the soap,[1] sodium oleate $(C_{17}H_{33} \cdot COONa)$ the polar $(-COONa)$ end, which is the hydrophilic

[1] A soap is a salt of certain of the fatty acids. See also page 34.

end of the molecule, has a greater cross-section than that of the non-polar ($C_{17}H_{33}-$) end. (Fig. 4.)

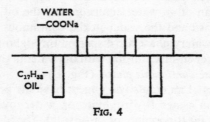

FIG. 4

If, owing to the number of soap molecules present, the oil water interface is increased, the bending of the interface will tend to take place thus:

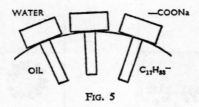

FIG. 5

Because the cross-section of the water-soluble portion of the molecule is greater than that of the fat-soluble portion, the tendency will be for the oil to form spheres enclosed by water, i.e. an oil-in-water emulsion will be formed. In the case of the calcium salts of the fatty acids the polar, hydrophilic end has a smaller cross-section than the non-polar, lipophilic end and these soaps tend to produce water-in-oil emulsions.

Oil-in-water emulsions are produced by acacia and other gums, sodium, potassium and ammonium soaps, casein, cetomacrogol 1000, egg yolk, glyceryl monostearate, Lanette Wax, etc. Water-in-oil emulsions are produced by wool fat, resins, beeswax and calcium soaps, etc.

There are important therapeutic differences between the two types of emulsions: for instance, water-soluble medicaments are generally more easily absorbed when the aqueous solution is in the continuous phase. This matter is more fully discussed on page 11 where ointments, pastes and creams are considered. It is important to remember that an emulsion can be diluted only with a material of the same nature as that of the continuous phase; that is to say, that a water-in-oil emulsion must be diluted with an oil and an oil-in-water emulsion must be diluted with an aqueous solution.

Colloidal-solutions may occasionally be encountered. In colloidal solutions, instead of individual molecules being dispersed throughout the solvent as in a true solution, the disperse phase consists of small aggregates of molecules. Strictly speaking, emulsions are colloidal solutions, but generally the term "colloidal solution" is reserved for those cases where the aggregates of molecules are very small. Frequently the aggregates of molecules all carry the same electrical charge, and since like charges repel, the colloidal state is maintained by the mutual repulsion of the charged aggregates.

In discussing the advantages and disadvantages of the various types of preparations it is probably most profitable to discuss them generally, under the headings of liquids, semi-solid and solid preparations.

THE LIQUID PREPARATIONS

The type of liquid preparation is frequently dictated by the nature of the medicament. Calamine is quite insoluble in anything but the mineral acids which cannot be applied to the skin and it is therefore generally prepared as a suspension. Cresol is sufficiently soluble only in solutions of soap and is usually dispensed as Cresol and Soap Solution B.P. In many cases, however, there is a choice of type of liquid preparation and therefore the general properties of each type must be discussed.

Aqueous solutions, solutions of medicaments in water, are usually applied as wet dressings. As a rule they are not used as paints because it is difficult to "wet" the skin with an aqueous solution of a drug. A notable exception to this is that solutions of silver nitrate in distilled water are widely used as paints. (It is possible to introduce wetting agents such as those used in photography which enable the silver nitrate solution to wet the skin more easily.) On the intact skin the tendency is for an aqueous solution to lie on the surface and not to penetrate. Aqueous solutions evaporate fairly slowly when exposed to the air. In the case of open wounds watery solutions of medicaments will mix freely with the blood serum and tissue fluid and the medicament will be easily absorbed from the watery medium. Sometimes, instead of a medicament being dispensed in distilled water, it is dispensed in a solution of a salt, e.g. because iodine is not very soluble in water it is dispensed in a solution of potassium iodide. For other reasons, aminacrine is sometimes dispensed in normal saline. Normal saline is isotonic with the blood fluid, that is to say it exerts the same osmotic pressure.[1] This means that when a delicate tissue is treated with such a solution there is no tendency for the tissue cells to become shrivelled up due to the osmotic pressure of the solution surrounding them being too high and thus causing the watery contents of the cell to pass out through the cell wall to the concentrated solution (plasmolysis); nor will the cells become distended with fluid because the osmotic pressure of the medium which surrounds them is low (plasmoptysis).

Apart from the effect of osmotic pressure on individual cells, it also affects the tissues in general. For instance, if a hypertonic solution is introduced into a wound there will be a tendency for fluid to flow from the tissues surrounding the wound, i.e. there will be an increase in the amount of lymph in the area of the wound. The effect is sometimes used therapeutically by employing a strong saline solution or a paste of magnesium sulphate in glycerin. If the solution of an antiseptic is isotonic with the tissue fluid, no such withdrawal of fluid will take place.

Certain drugs, notably the acridines, work best at a certain degree of acidity or alkalinity and these drugs are sometimes dispensed as buffered solutions. A buffered solution is one which changes its degree of acidity or alkalinity only very slowly when considerable quantities of free acid or alkali are added. By using suitable acids and salts the pH of a buffered solution may be adjusted to any desired value. Generally, when the acridines are dispensed, it is so arranged that the buffered solution is also isotonic with the tissue fluid. For convenience, solution tablets (Solvellae) are available for the preparation of buffered solutions, and are also employed for the preparation of stock solutions or solutions which have to be freshly made.

In contrast to the aqueous solutions are the spiritous solutions which are commonly prepared in ethyl alcohol or in iso-propyl alcohol. Iso-propyl alcohol has the advantage of being duty-free and non-intoxicating and many medicaments are more soluble in it than they are in ethyl alcohol. In a large number of preparations for external use Industrial Methylated Spirit may be used instead of ethyl alcohol. Details of the composition of Industrial Methylated

[1] Osmosis is the flow of water or other solvent through a semi-permeable membrane. A semi-permeable membrane is one which permits the passage of the solvent but not all of the dissolved substances. There is a tendency for solutions separated by a semi-permeable membrane to become equal in molecular concentration so that water will flow from a weaker to a stronger solution until the solutions are equal in concentration. The osmotic pressure is that pressure which must be applied to stop the flow of the solvent through the membrane, in other words the force with which the solvent tends to flow through the membrane. (See also footnote, page 45.)

Spirit which consists mainly of ethyl alcohol, but with other ingredients added, will be found on page 141. The spirituous solutions are generally painted on to the intact skin and allowed to dry. They wet the skin much more readily than the aqueous solutions and also evaporate much more rapidly. They are also employed as evaporating dressings. Sometimes a spirituous solution of one of the acridines is preferable to the aqueous solution as a wet dressing since the spirituous solution has a slightly stimulating and astringent effect and is less likely than is the aqueous solution to produce a macerated wound.

Other solutions, such as solutions in soap, in acetone or in ether, are generally dictated by the nature of the solute and are used because other solvents will not dissolve the particular medicament concerned.

THE SEMI-SOLID PREPARATIONS

The semi-solid preparations are the Creams, the Ointments and the Pastes. For convenience the Ointments and Creams will be considered together.

An ointment may be intended as a protection for the skin or, more commonly, be used as a base or vehicle for an active ingredient. The term "phase" has already been encountered on page 6. In a "double-phase" semi-solid two distinct physical forms may be identified. A "single-phase" semi-solid is homogenous.

Single Phase Greasy Semi-solids

In this category fall the vegetable, animal and mineral fats and greases. Mineral greases such as the paraffin hydrocarbons can be selected to produce a wide range of viscosities. They have the disadvantage that they tend to leave a persistent film that is greasy to the touch, but the advantage of protecting any medicament they contain from dissolving in water. Animal and vegetable fats are less greasy but they tend to become rancid over a period of time unless anti-oxidants are added.

Double Phase Greasy Semi-solids

The grease extracted from a sheep's wool will produce Wool Fat and Wool Alcohols when purified. These substances will take up considerable amounts of water to form water-in-oil emulsions. They may be used alone as a basis or may be mixed with paraffins. Although the emulsion so formed will still take up a certain quantity of water, it is not miscible with a large excess of water and it will not be washed away easily by water alone. The esters of polyhydric alcohols such as the monoglycerides, the diglycol esters and the sorbitol esters may also form emulsions of the water-in-oil type. These have the advantage that the characteristic "lanolin" odour and stickiness of the wool products are absent.

Single Phase Water-miscible Semi-solids

The group of chemicals called the polyethylene glycols (macrogols) fall into this category. Macrogols can be produced with a wide range of molecular weights, those of M.W. up to 700 being liquids; from 1,000 to 1,500 are semi-solids and from 4,000 to 6,000 waxy solids. The macrogols are colourless, odourless, non-toxic and have a neutral pH. This chemical series is similar in some respects to the paraffin series and its members have been called the Carbowaxes. These water-miscible bases are useful in cases where a superficial effect is required. Chemical incompatibility with the active ingredient may be a disadvantage in some cases.

Other forms of water-miscible semi-solids are the hydrogels. These are aqueous solutions in semi-solid form as a gel. The gel is formed by the use of a high concentration of a colloid and, because of the high water content, these preparations have a cooling effect on the skin. Protective colloids are formed by such compounds as methylcellulose and sodium carboxymethylcellulose, the carboxy-methylene polymers (Carbopols) and sodium alginate (related to the alginates used for cast-taking for appliances). The hydrogels present some difficulties during manufacture but make an ideal basis for water-soluble antiseptics.

Double Phase Water-miscible Semi-solids

These bases are oil-in-water Emulsions and Creams. They are water-miscible, washable and have a cooling effect due to the evaporation of water from the continuous phase. They are used to dispense water-soluble medicaments.

Oil-in-water emulsions are generally good media for the growth of bacteria and moulds. Because of this, a preservative such as 0·1 per cent Chlorocresol is usually added.

Emulgents to form these oil-in-water emulsions are of three types.

(*a*) Anionic, e.g. Sodium Lauryl Sulphate.

(*b*) Cationic, e.g. Cetrimide.

(*c*) Non-ionic, e.g. Cetomacrogol.

For an explanation of the terms aniomic, cationic and non-ionic and for a discussion of their properties see under "Detergents", page 33.

For most efficient use, the emulgents are usually used as an emulsifying wax, that is a mixture of emulgent and a thickener. For example Emulsifying Wax B.P. contains about 10 per cent sodium lauryl sulphate (an anionic emulgent) and 90 per cent cetostearyl alcohol mixed together with hot water to form a cream. Emulsifying Ointment B.P. contains 30 per cent Emulsifying Wax, 50 per cent White Soft Paraffin and 20 per cent Liquid Paraffin. Simple Cream B.P. contains 30 per cent Emulsifying Ointment with 70 per cent distilled water to which 0·1 per cent of chlorocresol is added as a preservative. The advantages of ointments and creams prepared with Emulsifying Wax are:

1. They are suitable vehicles for water-soluble medicaments.

2. The evaporation of water from the surface of the skin produces a cooling effect.

3. A lower percentage of active ingredient is required than is the case with a fatty ointment base.

4. The ointment can be rubbed into the skin leaving the surface free from greasiness.

5. Ointments prepared in this way are easily removed from skin and clothing.

The Pastes differ from the Ointments in that they are either prepared in a non-greasy base or in the fact that there is a very high proportion of powder mixed with a hydrocarbon such as soft or liquid paraffin. To be precise, most of the high strength salicylic ointments should be classed as pastes. Examples of the first type of paste commonly encountered in chiropody are Unna's Paste which is zinc oxide in a gelatin-glycerin base, and Morison's Paste (Magnesium Sulphate Paste) which is magnesium sulphate dispensed in a glycerin base. Lassar's Paste and Coal Tar and Zinc Paste are examples of the second type of paste. The last two are often spread on lint before application and, since they are stiff, they do not tend to clog the pores of the skin.

THE SOLID PREPARATIONS

The solid preparations which are used in chiropody may be divided into two groups; those which are applied to broken surfaces and to wounds, and those which are applied only to the intact skin.

Those which are applied to the broken skin are antibacterial preparations such as "Cicatrin" Powder (Calmic). Cicatrin contains antibiotics in powder form and is not self-sterilizing. This means that because the preparation is dry and in powder form it will not act on any bacteria which may contaminate it during storage. It must therefore be used and stored with care to avoid bacterial contamination.

The solid preparations which are used on the intact skin are the Dusting-powders. There are many variations of these powders, some official and many unofficial. A dusting-powder usually consists of a soothing or lubricant base with perhaps some active ingredient added. The materials which are used for the base include: Starch, Chalk, Magnesium Carbonate, Kaolin, Talc, Zinc Oxide and Zinc Stearate.

The following are the active ingredients most frequently encountered, with the strengths which are most commonly used:

1. Boric acid (not more than 5 per cent)—an antiseptic with, it is said, a specific action on *Bacterium foetidum*, the organism alleged to be responsible for the breakdown of sweat in certain cases of bromidrosis.

2. Salicylic acid (3–10 per cent)—astringent, antiseptic and fungicidal.

3. Alum (about 10 per cent)—a strong astringent and deodorant.

4. Benzocaine (about 10 per cent)—an active analgesic and antipruritic.

5. Calamine (up to 100 per cent)—soothing and absorbent.

6. Chlorphenesin (1 per cent)—fungicidal.

7. Camphor (1 per cent)—antipruritic and fungicidal.

8. Menthol (2 per cent)—antipruritic and fungicidal.

9. Phenol ($2\frac{1}{2}$ per cent)—sometimes used as an antiseptic.

10. Sodium borate (25 per cent)—antiseptic.

11. Sodium perborate (15 per cent)—antiseptic.

12. Sodium polymetaphosphate (5 per cent)—astringent and prophylactic against fungal infection.

13. Benzoin Tincture (10 per cent)—astringent and protective.

14. Thymol (1 per cent)—antiseptic and fungicidal.

15. Phenyl mercuric nitrate (0·2 per cent)—fungicidal.

16. Undecenoic acid (2 per cent) and the undecenoates (10 per cent)—fungicidal.

The official Dusting-powders, details of which will be found under the appropriate heading in Part Two are:

Chlorhexidine Dusting-powder B.P.C.
Chlorphenesin Dusting-powder B.P.C.
Hexachlorophane Dusting-powder B.P.C.
Talc Dusting-powder B.P.C.
Zinc and Salicylic Acid Dusting-powder B.P.C.
Zinc, Starch and Talc Dusting-powder B.P.C.
Zinc Undecenoate Dusting-powder B.P.C.

Unofficial dusting-powders are marketed under the various trade names and details of these will be found in the section of Monographs. The proprietary foot powders include:

"Pixcyl" (Fisons) see Coal Tar; "Mycil" (B.D.H.), "Tinaderm" (Glaxo), "S7" (Calmic) see Chlorphenesin; "Penotrane" (Ward, Blenkinsop) see Hydrargaphen; "Amoxal" (Smith & Nephew), "Episol" (Crookes), "Phytocil" (Wade) "Tineafax" (Burroughs Wellcome) see Undecenoic Acid.

Dusting-powders, especially those containing Kaolin, Talc and Diatomite should not be used on broken surfaces since these materials, being of natural origin may be contaminated with *Clostridium tetani* or *Clostridium welchii* in spite of precautions taken to sterilize the powder during manufacture. Another possible danger is that when dusting-powders come into contact with mucous surfaces granulomata may be produced.

PRESSURE PACKS

Pressurized packs, commonly referred to as aerosols, or aerosol dispensers, are now frequently used to dispense medicinal products. The product may vary in form including wound powders, spray-on bandages, dermatological applications, foams and creams.

The pack is made from metal, glass or plastic. The internal pressure is created by the incorporation of a propellant into the system. A great variety of propellants are in general use. They fall into two main categories: (1) compressed gases, some of which may be inflammable, e.g. propane, butanes, pentanes, hexanes, nitrogen, nitrous oxide and carbon dioxide: (2) non-inflammable halogenated hydrocarbons. This group is the one generally chosen and there are so many with complex chemical names that they have been given numbers for identification, e.g. Propellant 12—difluorodichloromethane.

The choice of propellant is made with consideration to the following factors: inflammability, vapour pressure, solubility and compatibility with the product to be sprayed, also the liability to corrode the valve, nozzle, spray, or container.

Pressurised packs are expensive to manufacture. They comprise a container fitted with a dip tube, valve and accelerator nozzle. The disadvantage of expense can be balanced against the advantages of application. Pressure packs make it possible to apply a very thin film of a medicament without resorting to the use of swabs of cotton wool or other methods of "painting". The sterility of the product is well maintained. It is often difficult, however, to confine the spray to a defined area and a certain amount of product is transferred to the atmosphere, and to the surrounding objects. This is particularly noticeable with sprays of Friars' Balsam and similar "sticky" products.

Examples of aerosols used in chiropody are "Rikospray Balsam", "Nobecutane" and "Octaflex".

CHAPTER II

THE ACTION OF MEDICAMENTS

ABSORBENTS

AN *Absorbent* takes up excretions from the body, e.g.: pus, lymph and serum from lesions, or sweat in the case of hyperidrosis.

Dusting-powders, which are of course extensively used in the treatment of hyperidrosis, should not be regarded as being absorbent. Too little of the powder is used to warrant such a concept. The most important function of dusting-powders is lubrication and they reduce friction on the skin surface: they may have other functions according to their "active ingredient", see page 12.

The absorbents which are used in chiropody include cotton dressings such as lint, gauze and cotton wool. A dressing called "Melolin XA" has been produced which consists of a non-adherent plastic film of melolin, which is non-absorbent, over gauze which is absorbent. There is also an absorbent dressing "Calgitex" which contains calcium alginate. This is primarily used as an absorbable haemostatic. Kaolin Poultice, in addition to being a means of applying moist heat, has a marked absorbent action and, since it contains a large percentage of kaolin which is highly absorbent, takes up pus, lymph, serum, etc., from the wounds to which it is applied. Glycerin is highly hygroscopic, that is to say, it has a strong affinity for water and will absorb moisture from the tissues.

ANALGESICS, ANAESTHETICS AND ANTIPRURITICS

An *Analgesic* is a medicament which lessens and relieves pain.
An *Anaesthetic* is a medicament which lessens sensitivity to pain.

It will be seen from a study of these definitions that while all anaesthetics are *per se* analgesics, a drug which, for instance, relieves congestion, may act as an analgesic without being anaesthetic.

Anaesthetics act directly on the nervous system but their mode of action is uncertain. It is thought that the effects may be produced in the myelinated fibres, at the nodes of Ranvier where it is known that ion exchanges occur. Anaesthetics act on all nervous tissue so that impulses are prevented from (*a*) arising and (*b*) passing. The main

15

problem in applying surface anaesthetics in chiropody is to bring the anaesthetic into contact with the nerve endings. Such drugs as benzocaine, lignocaine ("Xylodase") and amethocaine hydrochloride are effective only when they are brought into direct contact with the pain nerve endings. Thus these drugs are very disappointing in nail groove work and when applied topically as a solution prior to the removal of the nucleus of a painful corn, but they are sometimes very effective when they are applied in an ointment base as a dressing to neurovascular corns. Ethyl chloride acts by evaporating rapidly and causing the tissues to freeze and thus rendering them insensitive to pain. However, it also hardens the tissues and since the pain of thawing is often worse than the original pain the use of this technique has been virtually discontinued in chiropody.

Local anaesthetics may also be introduced into the tissues by means of injection. Infiltration anaesthesia is a technique whereby the nerve endings are anaesthetized by direct exposure to the drug. Since local anaesthetics also prevent the transmission of impulses along the nerve-fibre the tissues may be infiltrated round an area, giving a ring block, or nerves may be anaesthesized along the course of the nerve. For topical use adrenaline is sometimes added to a local anaesthetic to cause vaso-constriction and the localization of the anaesthetic and prolongation of its action. This is contra-indicated in chiropody practice. The local anaesthetics are destroyed mainly by the liver and the rate at which they are destroyed is a major factor in determining the safety of their use.

There is a group of drugs which act as rubefacients, relieving congestion, which also have some direct action on the nerves and the nerve endings. Heat acts in this way and also the group of medicaments which includes menthol, camphor, clove oil, methyl salicylate, etc. These agents produce mild inflammation of the skin. There are many theories about how they act and their mode of action must be regarded as uncertain. It is certain that the psychological effect is important. These agents act by removing the cause of the pain as well as having some action on the nerves themselves.

An *Antipruritic* is a medicament which relieves itching.

The term "antipruritic" means "against itching". The benzocaine-amethocaine group of drugs are antipruritic and are frequently employed to relieve itching. They act upon the nerves and nerve endings. The rubefacients are employed in order to relieve itching in chilblains, by clearing the congestion in the area, and promoting the absorption of the static metabolites. Other medicaments, such as

Calamine Lotion, Kaolin Powder and Witch Hazel Lotion allay itching by producing a cooling effect on the skin. The application of an alkaline lotion, such as Lime Water, to the skin will often have the effect of reducing itching. The antihistamines are frequently used when treating pruritis, although they are not strictly classed as anti-pruritics. They form a group of drugs which act by preventing histamine reaching its site of action. Mepyramine maleate: "Anthisan" (May & Baker), is useful in allergic pruritis and 10 per cent Crotamiton in an ointment base, "Eurax" (Geigy), is a very effective non-specific antipruritic.

ANHIDROTICS

An *Anhidrotic* is a medicament which, applied externally, reduces the flow of sweat.

The action of the anhidrotics is often described as being "astringent". The use of the term "astringent" is discussed below, and it will be seen that reduction in the flow of perspiration has come to be regarded as part of astringent action. Exactly how the anhidrotics produce their effect is not known, but it is certain that they do not all act in the same way. Some have cooling action, and thus invoke the heat-regulating mechanism of the body; alcohol acts in this way but is also an astringent. Some powders have an astringent action on the skin. These include salicylic acid, tannic acid, alum and sodium polymetaphosphate.

It seems probable that, rather than reducing the amount of sweat produced, the chief action of many of the anhidrotics is that of preventing the sweat from having a deleterious effect on the skin, either by altering the texture of the epidermis and so improving its water-resisting properties, or by anti-wetting action. Formalin may work in this way.

Medicaments which are used as anhidrotics include alcohol, alum, aluminium acetate, copper sulphate, formalin, silver nitrate and zinc oxide. Salicylic acid, camphor, menthol and tannic acid are used as ingredients of anhidrotic lotions and powders.

ANTIBIOTICS

The term antibiotic is reserved for substances, produced in culture during the growth of certain fungi or bacteria, or to similar substances produced synthetically, which inhibit the vital processes of micro-organisms other than the species producing them.

There are now hundreds of known antibiotics although only a proportion of them have been developed for therapeutic use. The development of antibiotics since 1941 has been a most important development in medicine but it became at one time one of the most abused forms of drug therapy. The prescription of antibiotics is now controlled by the Therapeutic Substances Act 1956, but the Act only limits those who may prescribe the drug and not the uses to which they may be put. The dangers in the use of antibiotics may affect both the patient and the community.

Unless an infection is completely cleared and all the organisms killed, resistant strains may emerge which may be disseminated to the danger of public health. The risk of infection with antibiotic-resistant organisms is particularly great in hospitals and elaborate steps are taken to minimize such risks.

Other problems associated with the use of antibiotics are:
  (i) Cross-resistance between different antibiotics.
 (ii) Sensitization which may occur especially if topical treatment is used.
(iii) Supra-infection, an example of which is that if some of the organisms normally found in the mouth are supressed by the use of a wide-spectrum antibiotic the antibiotic-resistant species *Candida* will multiply in the mouth causing the infection known as "thrush".

The main problem with the increased use of antibiotics is the emergence of resistant strains of "super-microbes". Chiropodists working in hospitals will sometimes find that topical antibiotics are used but only those antibiotics which are not commonly used systematically are used in this way. Neomycin sulphate, bacitracin, sodium fucidate and, very occasionally, the tetracyclines are used topically (see Antibiotics used Topically in Part II). Griseofulvin is used systemically in the treatment of fungal infections and nystatin and pecilocin are used topically for the same purpose.

The great advantage of the use of antibiotics is that while they do have certain systemic effects, they interfere with vital processes of micro-organisms and fungi and do not affect the tissues in general. Modern developments in complex organic substances such as Clio-quinol and Polynoxylin have provided acceptable substitutes for the topical antibiotics in the treatment of ulcerations of the feet associated with systemic disorders and it may well be that further developments will take place in the future. The topical antibiotics remain the most useful antibacterial agents available for application in powder form.

ANTI-INFLAMMATORY AGENTS

An *Anti-inflammatory* agent is one which reduces inflammation; they
have previously been termed "antiphlogistics". The anti-inflammatory agents which are used in chiropody fall under three main
headings: (1) the rubefacients, (2) heat, (3) cold.

1. The rubefacients act by stimulating a mild inflammation over
a wide area and thus relieve congestion and stasis.

2. Heat is a manifestation of kinetic energy of molecules. The
molecules of all substances are in a state of oscillation and an increase in the rate of oscillation manifests itself as a rise in temperature.
Heat energy can be transmitted from molecule to molecule directly
by conduction, or it may be converted into electro-magnetic radiations which may be absorbed and reconverted into heat energy.

The temperature of a substance and the quantity of heat it contains are not one and the same. The unit of heat-quantity is the calorie.
One calorie will raise the temperature of one gramme of copper
through ten degrees centigrade. Thus copper requires less heat to
raise its temperature than does water and the specific heat (i.e. the
number of calories required to raise one gramme of a substance
through one degree centigrade) of copper is less than that of water.
It requires 1·25 calories to raise the temperature of one gramme of
tissue through one degree centigrade; the specific heat of the tissues
is very high and the quantity of heat applied is very important. Since
water also has a high specific heat a foot-bath is a good method of
applying a large quantity of heat.

The effect of raising the temperature of the tissues is to invoke the
heat regulating mechanism of the body. The body tends to remain
at a constant temperature and does so by controlling the amount of
heat it loses to the surroundings. To increase the amount of heat loss
(a) the secretion of the sweat is stimulated so that heat is lost by the
evaporation of the sweat from the skin, and (b) the superficial blood
vessels also become dilated so that there is an increase in the amount
of heat lost from the body by radiation. When the temperature of the
tissues is raised the arterioles, venules and capillaries become dilated
and there is an increase in the amount of blood passing through a
vessel in a given time. In addition to there being an increase in the
rate of flow there is also an increase in the capillary blood pressure.
The interchange of fluid between the capillaries and the tissue depends

on the physical balance between the outward pressure exerted by the hydrostatic pressure of the blood in the capillaries and the inward pressure exerted by the osmotic attraction of the proteins which are unable to diffuse through the vessel wall. When the hydrostatic pressure in the capillaries is raised due to the action of heat there will be an increase in the amount of fluid pushed out into the tissue spaces.

The speeding up of the rate of blood flow will also have an effect on the amount of oxygen and carbon dioxide in the blood. At very low temperatures the metabolic rate of the tissues is reduced almost to nothing and therefore little oxygen is used up and the amount of oxygen contained in the venous blood is high. A slight increase in temperature will result in an increase in tissue metabolism without a corresponding increase, or without a sufficient increase, in the rate of blood flow and the amount of oxygen in the venous blood will be low. At about 43° C. the rate of the blood flow is increased so much that in spite of a high rate of tissue metabolism the venous blood is nearly indistinguishable from arterial blood. With the increase in circulation due to an increase in temperature the tissues are exposed to more blood per unit of time and also the activity of the leucocytes is increased.

The most important therapeutic effect of heat is the increase in the rate of blood flow but, in estimating the value of heat in any inflammatory condition, it must be remembered that there is an increase in exudation of fluid from the vessels, so causing a local oedema, which in certain cases may interfere with the circulation. A mild application of heat will often be beneficial when an intensive one may harm the capillary blood vessels and cause considerable exudation of fluid and congestion.

Heat can be applied in the form of:

(a) *Hot fomentations and poultices.* Lint fomentations are rarely used in chiropody. The quantity of heat available is small and they have to be renewed frequently. Kaolin Poultice B.P. has the advantage of absorbing discharges from lesions and it also has the advantage of acting as an insulator against heat loss. Hot fomentations and poultices are moist forms of heat and cause the skin to become macerated and weakened and, since they are localized in their action, they are useful for causing pus to "point" and so establish drainage.

(b) *Hot foot-baths.* Hot foot-baths are generally of water but paraffin wax and sand are sometimes used. The action of hot foot-baths is diffuse and they have general as well as local effects. The quantity of heat available is large, especially in the case of water foot-baths, and the temperature of the water can be kept comparatively low at about 46° C. "Foot-baths" of paraffin wax may be used where a higher temperature is required; a temperature of 51–55° C. is tolerated in a paraffin wax bath but not in a water bath. The evaporation of sweat and loss of heat by radiation from the skin are reduced by the solidification of the inner layers of wax on the skin, the wax acting as an insulator preventing the loss of absorbed heat. Wax baths are particularly useful in cases of foot strain.

(c) *Visible and infra-red radiations.* Special apparatus is required for the application of heat by these methods. The electric heating pad gives mainly non-penetrating radiations over a diffuse area. It is a convenient method for home use by the patient. The black body infra-red generator gives long and short rays some of which penetrate to the subcutaneous tissues but the majority are absorbed by the surface tissues. The incandescent light bulb or radiant heat lamp gives penetrating radiations most of which are transmitted by the surface tissues to be absorbed by the subcutaneous and deeper tissues. The advantages of using the black body generator or the radiant heat lamp are that nothing has to come into direct contact with the skin or with any lesion of the skin. There is no pressure on the tissues, and medicaments may be applied while the treatment is taking place. However, they can be applied conveniently only for short periods of up to half an hour at a time. The application of infra-red and radiant heat radiations appears to have a marked sedative effect and to relieve pain to a considerable degree.

Heat may be used as a rubefacient but is contra-indicated where there is a serious deficiency in the circulation, either arterial or venous, where the heat-regulating mechanism of the body is not functioning properly or where the appreciation of heat is diminished as in cases of diabetic neuropathy.

3. Cold has the reverse effect of heat in the fact that it diminishes the flow of blood and the exudation of fluid from the blood vessels. It is therefore contra-indicated when there is bacterial infection or when the circulation is already poor.

Cold can be applied in the form of:
(a) Cold compresses.
(b) Cold foot-baths.
(c) Ice packs.
(d) Evaporating lotions.

Corticosteroids are used in other fields of medicine as topical anti-inflammatory agents but they are available on prescription only (S4B). These are very powerful anti-inflammatory agents but they tend to mask the symptoms without curing the cause. The corticosteroids have important side-effects and it is often necessary to modify therapeutic procedures when treating patients who are receiving these drugs systemically. Basically, they suppress the normal processes of inflammation thereby reducing the natural defences against both infection and trauma. See also page 67.

ANTISEPTICS

The word "Antiseptic" is a popular term and does not have a precise meaning. It is taken to include all drugs which either kill or inhibit pathogenic micro-organisms. The word "Disinfectant" is also a popular term applied to all agents which kill micro-organisms but is generally used when the agent is being applied to an inanimate object.

The technical terms which have a precise meaning are:

"Bactericide"—an agent which kills bacteria.

"Bacteriostatic"—an agent which inhibits the growth of bacteria and prevents them from multiplying, without actually killing them.

"Germicide"—an agent which kills pathogenic micro-organisms. It is, however, a non-specific term and therefore best avoided.

"Virucide"—an agent which kills viruses.

"Fungicide"—an agent which kills fungi.

"Fungistatic"—an agent which inhibits the growth of fungi.

"Parasiticide"—which in its widest sense, embraces anything which will kill an animal or a vegetable parasite, is used particularly for drugs which kill animal parasites such as *Sarcoptes* and *Pediculus*.

The use of antiseptics is a fundamental study in chiropody and the application of antiseptics to various conditions is discussed extensively in later chapters. Before considering the application of antiseptics certain theoretical factors must be discussed.

Antiseptic action depends on:

(1) The **Time** during which the antiseptic is in contact with the organisms, the **Temperature** and the **Concentration** of the antiseptic.

(2) The nature of the organisms on which the antiseptic is acting.

(3) The nature of the substrate, that is the surroundings in which the antiseptic has to act.

When considering bacterial activity, it is not sufficient to say that a 1 per cent solution of a certain antiseptic will kill *Staphylococcus aureus*, what must be said is that a 1 per cent solution of the antiseptic will kill this organism in so many minutes at such a temperature in a stated substrate. Bactericides do not act instantaneously but require time in which to function and this point cannot be stressed too strongly. Generally speaking, the weaker the concentration of any antiseptic the longer will be the time required to kill the bacteria. Time, temperature and concentration are linked together, in that the greater the concentration, and the higher the temperature, the shorter is the time required to kill the micro-organisms, and vice versa. This holds true only within certain limits since there is a minimum concentration required before the bacteria will be killed and, if this concentration is not reached, the antiseptic may act only as a bacteriostatic or, if the concentration is very small, it may have no effect at all. Since, in chiropody, there is generally no opportunity of altering the temperature at which the antiseptic action takes place, it may be considered that:

$$C^n \propto \frac{1}{t}$$

where C = the concentration of the bactericide,
  t = the time for a stated kill,
and n = the dilution coefficient.

Thus, for a given bactericide under stated conditions n may be determined. It is found that the phenols have a high dilution coefficient, i.e. phenolic activity is quickly removed by dilution, and the surface active agents have a low coefficient.

A given antiseptic does not have the same effect on all micro-organisms. Indeed some antiseptics are very highly selective and have a marked action on certain groups of organisms at quite low concentration and little or no effect on others. Crystal violet, for example, is quite effective against Gram-positive[1] organisms but has no effect on Gram-negative organisms. The range of bacteria against which a drug is effective is known as its antibacterial spectrum.

The nature of the substrate is important since many antiseptics are inhibited by the presence of reactive organic material such as blood, tissue, etc., or by the presence of pus. This is particularly important when choosing antiseptics for use on intact skin, on fresh wounds, on septic wounds or on ulcers.

THE CHOICE OF AN ANTISEPTIC

"If you can measure that of what you speak, and can express it

[1] See footnote page 29.

by a number, you know something of your subject: but if you cannot measure it, your knowledge is meagre and unsatisfactory." These words, written by a physicist, Lord Kelvin, sum up the scientists' preference to evaluate all phenomena in terms of numbers, a preference which is shared by many members of the general public. From the earliest days, even before the germ theory of disease was finally accepted, attempts were made to evaluate antiseptics in terms of numbers so that it could be said that antiseptic A was twice as efficient as antiseptic B and three and a half times as efficient as antiseptic C.

The action of an antiseptic depends on time, temperature and concentration and these factors are taken into consideration in the test devised by Rideal and Walker in 1903 and which, with slight modifications, is still widely used today. In brief, the Rideal-Walker test consists of a comparison under standard conditions between the concentration of the antiseptic under test with the concentration of phenol required to kill a standard strain of *Salmonella typhosa* in a given time. The Rideal-Walker co-efficient is the highest dilution of the antiseptic under test not killing in five minutes but killing in seven-and-a-half minutes divided by the dilution of phenol which will do the same. Thus if a 1–300 dilution of an antiseptic kills *S. typhosa* in seven-and-a-half minutes but not in five minutes and 1–100 dilution of Phenol does the same then the Rideal-Walker co-efficient of that antiseptic is 300 divided by 100, i.e. 3. The test is carried out at a standard temperature of 15–18° C.

The Rideal-Walker test does yield a numerical answer, but the limitations of this and similar tests are obvious. First, the test-organism is not commonly encountered in chiropody and because an antiseptic is three times as effective as phenol against *S. typhosa*, it is not necessarily three times as effective as phenol against *Staphylococcus aureus*. It is quite easy to substitute the latter as the test organism, and this is done frequently, and the test yields information of interest and value to those who require an antiseptic to deal with that organism. It is important to remember that the Rideal-Walker co-efficient always refers to the action of the antiseptic on *Salmonella typhosa*. When another test organism is substituted the result may be described as "the Phenol coefficient against *S. aureus*", etc. Second, there is the choice of phenol for a comparison. Phenol has the advantage of being a definite chemical compound and is therefore easily defined, and it is stable and cheap. It is also fairly uniformly effective against most of the common pathogens. But the phenol coefficient of an antiseptic which is unrelated to phenol, and kills bacteria by an entirely different mechanism, may be very misleading. Third, there is the fact that the test takes place *in vitro*, that is under laboratory conditions, and not under conditions which will obtain in practice. In the Rideal-Walker test the action takes place in the absence of organic material and this further detracts from its practical value.

Other methods have been devised for overcoming the objection to the Rideal-Walker and similar tests but the results are never simple to interpret. Tests in the laboratory will give valuable indications as to the possible effects of the antiseptic *in vivo*, but the true value of an antiseptic can be finally assessed only on the basis of practical experience and observation.

In selecting an antiseptic for a given purpose a number of factors have to be taken into consideration.

1. *The nature of the infecting organism*. It has already been pointed out that many antiseptics are highly selective in their action, and if, for example, a wound was thought to be infected with *Pseudomonas pyocyanea*, a Gram-negative organism, then an antiseptic which is effective against Gram-negative organisms must be selected. This question is dealt with further under the heading of Treatment of Sepsis.

2. *The nature of the substrate*. An antiseptic which is effective on the unbroken skin may be useless in the presence of blood and other readily reactive organic material.

3. *Tissue toxicity of the antiseptic*. Bacterial cells and tissue cells are very similar in their structure and antiseptics which have a chemical action, such as oxidation, protein precipitation, etc., will affect both bacterial and tissue cells.

Certain antiseptics such as the acridines, and to a lesser extent the other aniline dyes, act as bacteriostatics by interfering in various ways with the metabolism of the bacteria. These antiseptics, therefore, generally have a very low tissue toxicity. There is another very important aspect of the toxic effects of antiseptics.

4. *The effect of the antiseptic on phagocytosis and the natural defence mechanism of the body*. Sir Alexander Fleming performed a series of experiments to demonstrate the effect of some types of antiseptics on the bactericidal power of the blood. Equal volumes of blood infected with *Staphylococci* or *Streptococci*, and various dilutions of chemical antiseptics in normal saline were mixed together, run into slide cells and incubated. Some of the results are indicated below. Normal human blood will kill off 95 per cent of the bacteria

present but, since leucocytes are more susceptible to the action of chemical antiseptics, certain concentrations of antiseptics remove the bactericidal power of the blood by killing the leucocytes without giving any protection against bacteria as compensation for this loss.

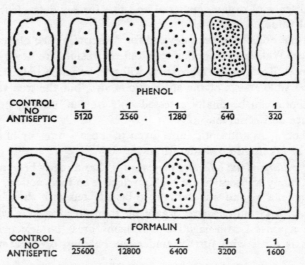

PHENOL

| CONTROL NO ANTISEPTIC | $\frac{1}{5120}$ | $\frac{1}{2560}$ | $\frac{1}{1280}$ | $\frac{1}{640}$ | $\frac{1}{320}$ |

FORMALIN

| CONTROL NO ANTISEPTIC | $\frac{1}{25600}$ | $\frac{1}{12800}$ | $\frac{1}{6400}$ | $\frac{1}{3200}$ | $\frac{1}{1600}$ |

FIG. 6. Sir Alexander Fleming's experiment—slide cells after incubation. The black dots represent bacterial colonies. The results show that concentrations of phenol between 1–500 and 1–600, and formalin 1–6.500 deprive the blood of its bactericidal power without giving protection in compensation.

5. *The power of the penetration of the antiseptic*. All chiropodists are familiar with the result of painting the skin surface with Silver Nitrate. A very shallow black coagulum is formed. By precipitating the tissue chlorides the silver nitrate forms an impermeable barrier of silver chloride which prevents any further penetration of the former. Some antiseptics, especially the salts of the heavy metals, which act by precipitating cell protein, also have the effect of preventing their own penetration.

6. *The surface tension of the antiseptic solution*. This affects the ability of the antiseptic to penetrate into the cracks and crevices of the skin or the wound. Antiseptics dispensed in solutions having a low surface tension will "wet" a surface to which they are applied more easily than those dispensed in solutions having a high surface tension.

Surface tension has another important effect on the action of an antiseptic. If an antiseptic has a low surface tension there will be a tendency for the material in solution to collect at the interface between the solution and any particulate matter. If bacteria form the only particulate matter in contact with the solution this is an advantage, but if there is much extraneous particulate matter present, the antiseptic will concentrate at all interfaces and may be removed entirely from the solution. This surface absorption is the reason why solutions of surface acting antiseptics should not be re-used.

7. *Detergent action.* Since bacteria are frequently imbedded in grease and other material, antiseptics which possess the property of emulsifying or dissolving greases and removing debris are useful when dirty or greasy surfaces have to be disinfected.

8. *The velocity of the antiseptic.* It has already been stated that the speed with which an antiseptic acts depends on its temperature and the concentration. Low concentrations of certain antiseptics function fairly rapidly due to the nature of their action, e.g. the oxidizing agents and the protein precipitants. This quality is useful in certain instances; in other cases it may be desirable to employ an antiseptic which exerts a fairly mild action for a long period of time. This contrast will be seen between the choice of antiseptic made for pre-operative use, when a quickly acting agent is an advantage, or for post-operative use, when a mild, lasting action is desirable.

9. *Solubility.* Surface acting agents act at the bacterial cell wall where they become absorbed. The highest absorption is achieved in an aqueous medium. It is, therefore, an advantage for an antiseptic to be soluble in water.

10. *Homogenicity.* An antiseptic should not vary in composition from time to time or from sample to sample. Acriflavine, which is a variable mixture of two chemicals, is an example of an antiseptic which is not homogenous. Cresol with Soap Solution B.P. may vary in its germicidal activity according to the type of soap with which it is prepared. It is also important that a solution of an antiseptic should be homogenous in the sense that each sample of the solution should be the same as every other sample. There should, for instance, be no excess concentration of the medicament at the top or the bottom of the bottle. Unfortunately, preferential concentration in a liquid preparation is sometimes unavoidable so that all liquid preparations should be thoroughly shaken before use unless specific instructions are given to the contrary.

11. *Stability.* It is a great advantage if an antiseptic is stable and will store well. The chlorine antiseptics and solutions of Hydrogen Peroxide are unstable and have to be stored very carefully or be freshly prepared.

12. *Corrosiveness.* If an antiseptic is to come into contact with instruments or any metal objects it is important that it should not be corrosive.

13. *Odour.* Some antiseptics have an unpleasant odour and others, notably the chloroxylenol-terpineol preparations, have a slight but very persistent and very clinging odour which may be objectionable to some people.

14. *Colour.* If the area has to be painted, it must be clearly seen, and it is important to know that it has actually been painted with antiseptic, it is an advantage for the antiseptic to be coloured. On the other hand it is a nuisance when an antiseptic obliterates the skin to such an extent that the progress of lesions cannot be observed.

15. *Cost.* If a large amount of antiseptic is required, for instance in a foot-bath, certain antiseptics may be ruled out on the grounds of expense.

The antiseptics commonly used in chiropody may be grouped as follows:

The Oxidizing agents

E.g. hydrogen peroxide, potassium permanganate. This group is rapid in action but by nature of their action they are extremely toxic to the affected tissues. However, they cannot penetrate very far owing to a self-created barrier. The oxidizing agents are ineffective if much organic material is present.

The Halogens

E.g. chlorine, iodine. These are rapid in action but are very irritant to the tissues. Their action is abolished if much organic material is present but they are very effective when this is not the case. Hypochlorites, e.g. calcium hypochlorite ("Eusol") and sodium hypochlorite ("Dakin's solution") are useful antiseptics of low tissue toxicity.

The Salts and Compounds of the Heavy Metals

E.g. silver, mercury, etc. These are slow in their action and cause considerable damage to the tissues. They are largely inactivated by the presence of organic material. Their germicidal efficiency varies from moderate to very good.

Alcohols

These form a large group of antiseptics of variable bactericidal efficiency. The alcohols are largely inactivated in the presence of proteins. They are rapid in their action; some are moderately toxic to the tissues, others are more toxic.

Coal Tar Derivatives

These all have a high dilution coefficient, that is they are effective in low concentrations. They include the following:

(a) Phenol is only moderately efficient as a bactericide and is fairly rapid in its action. Its tissue toxicity prohibits its use as a wound dressing.

(b) Cresol, as Cresol and Soap B.P. ("Lysol"), is highly toxic to the tissues. It loses some of its effect in the presence of organic material and is moderately rapid in its action.

(c) The halogenated cresols, e.g. Chloroxylenol Solution B.P. ("Dettol"), Hycolin. These are only slightly toxic to the tissues and are moderately rapid in their action. They lose much of their efficiency in the presence of organic material.

(d) The triphenylmethane dyes, e.g. crystal violet, brilliant green. These lose much of their efficiency in the presence of organic material and are slow in their action. Brilliant green is moderately toxic to the tissues and crystal violet somewhat less toxic. They are selective in their action.

(e) The acridine dyes, e.g. proflavine, aminacrine, etc. These are slow in action but are virtually non-toxic to the tissues and do not impair leucocytic activity. Their action is not greatly affected by the presence of organic material. They are selective in their action but are very effective against certain types of bacteria.

Cationic Surface-Active Agents

Cationic surface-active agents, e.g. cetrimide, domiphen bromide, benzalkonium chloride, chlorhexidine, have a low tissue toxicity, a wide spectrum of activity and are active in the presence of organic matter. Chlorhexidine is particularly useful since it combines a low dilution coefficient with the other general properties of the group. Sodium nitrite must be added to the solution if it is used for instrument storage so that corrosion is prevented.

Hypertonic solutions of various salts kill bacteria by virtue of their osmotic action. They withdraw water from the protoplasm of an organism.

Gram-negative, Gram-positive: Gram staining is a method whereby bacteria are divided into two classes according to whether or not they take up certain stains. For details of technique the reader is referred to a textbook of bacteriology. The significance of Gram staining is that it is closely linked with the effect of certain antiseptics on bacteria. Gram-negative organisms are especially resistant to certain antiseptics.

ASTRINGENTS

Classically, an *Astringent* was defined as a medicament which caused a shrinkage of the cells of a mucous membrane. The term was also applied to costive medicines. The use of astringents in nasal and ophthalmic work led to an extension of the definition to include a medicament which led to the arrest of a discharge. Many of the medicaments which act as astringents on mucous membranes also have an effect on the skin. This effect has not been clearly analysed but perhaps the best examples of the use of astringents on the skin are the "after-shave lotion" and the "enlarged pore-closer". Goodman suggests that the application of these lotions causes a mild inflammation of the skin and that the apparent tightening of skin is not due to any contraction of the tissue but to a mild inflammatory oedema. The true astringents, in the classical sense, when applied to the skin, are found to produce an apparent diminution in the flow of sweat. Because drugs labelled "astringents" have this effect when applied to the skin, their action, when so applied, is described, quite unjustifiably, as "astringency". Thus medicaments which produce on the skin effects similar to those of the true astringents, even though they exert no astringent action on mucous membrane, are described as astringents. At the present time the terms "astrict", "astringency" and "astringent" have very wide but rather confused meanings. Again, formalin, because it is used as a treatment for warts, has been called a caustic, although it neither precipitates protein nor destroys cells.

It is easy to condemn a word but quite another matter to find an alternative to put in its place. Therefore until a better word can be found the word "astringent" must continue in use to describe the group of medicaments which produce these effects on the skin. It must be clearly understood that the term "astringency" is used to describe the effect on the epidermis of those drugs which cause a shrinkage of the cells of mucous membranes and that the term "astringent" has been extended to include those drugs which, when applied to the skin, produce the same effect as true astringents.

The true astringents act on the mucous membrane by:

(*a*) Precipitating the cell proteins, e.g. the salts of the heavy metals. The medicaments in this group of astringents are often dilute strengths of the caustics and it is always difficult to define the point where astringency ends and causticity begins.

(*b*) Withdrawing fluid from the tissues, e.g. glycerin and the higher strengths of alcohol.

The effects of these groups on the skin varies. The first group has the effect of hardening the skin and apparently reducing the flow of sweat, or of making the skin more resistant to the effect of sweat. The second group has an effect on the skin which is probably nothing to do with their property of withdrawing water from the tissues. Glycerin acts as an emollient and alcohol has a cooling effect due to evaporation from the surface of the skin.

It is well known that cold water exerts an action on the skin similar to that of the astringents. Much the same sensations can be produced by an after-shave lotion and by plunging the face into a bowl of cold water. Hence cold exerts an astringent action and substances such as alcohol, which evaporates readily from the skin and so invokes the heat regulating mechanism of the body, act as astringents in a similar way. Alcohol is also a protein precipitant. The action of formalin is not well understood but it seems that it has some specific effect on the cell membrane, causing hardening and shrinking of the cell. Medicaments which are used in chiropody as astringents in the widest sense include preparations containing: salicylic acid, tannic acid, alcohol, alum, silver nitrate, Compound Benzoin Tincture, bismuth carbonate, calamine, chromium trioxide, copper sulphate, ferric chloride, formaldehyde, witch hazel, lead subacetate solution, trinitrophenol, zinc chloride, zinc stearate, glycerin and crystal violet. The individual properties of these medicaments are discussed in Part Two.

CAUSTICS

A *Caustic* is a medicament which destroys organic tissue. This is the widest possible definition of a caustic and covers a number of drugs having widely different actions on the skin. The word "escharotic" is better avoided since the definition of "eschar" varies quite widely. Some authorities regard an eschar as being the result of the application of a strong mineral acid, others as the exfoliated tissue produced by such caustics as salicylic acid, and yet others as precipitated protein which is produced by the action of such drugs as silver nitrate. Support for all three of these definitions will be found in current medical dictionaries. Another word which is used to describe a certain type of caustic is "keratolytic". This implies a drug having a specific action on the keratinized cells of the stratum corneum.

The action of many of the caustics is very complex and, in a majority of cases, imperfectly understood. Most caustics act by precipitating the protein of cell protoplasm but it must be remembered that in the skin we are dealing with cells of widely differing morphology and it is not possible to conceive, for example, one of the salts of the heavy metals "precipitating the protein" of the cells of the already keratinized stratum corneum. When considering the action of the caustics the action of the medicament must be related to the type of cell upon which it is to act. Certain medicaments will act in one way if they are applied to the skin where some stratum corneum has been left and in another way if they are applied to the skin where the stratum corneum has been removed. The medicaments which have an action on the stratum corneum, the keratolytics, act by breaking the side salt linkages between the long chains of the keratin molecules. This allows molecules of water to penetrate between the long keratin chains, causing maceration and an increase in the bulk of the tissues. The breaking up of the keratinized layer also allows the medicament itself to penetrate to the deeper layer and to act upon the non-keratinized cells. The medicaments which act in this way are the weak acids such as the chlor-acetic acids and salicylic acid, and the alkalis potassium and sodium hydroxide. The sulphides of many metals, notably barium and sodium, also act upon keratin but these are rarely used in chiropody. It is stressed that the action of the keratolytics is not to destroy the stratum corneum but only to soften and macerate it. Consider the case of a wart which has "broken down" under the action of salicylic acid: nearly always, before the sloughed-out ulcer is encountered, a thickened cap of intact tissue has to be removed. The caustic has destroyed the non-keratinized cells after penetrating the horny layer, but the latter is still intact. It is on this point, of course, that difficulty is encountered with proprietary corn paints and wart "solvents"—the coagulum resulting from the action of salicylic acid which these remedies usually contain, must be removed, and skilfully removed, if the patient is to obtain relief and infection is to be avoided. The caustics can never take the place of the adequate removal of callus with a knife; they must be used in conjunction with, and not as a substitute for, careful operating.

The action of caustics on non-keratinized cells is in a large number of cases, that of precipitating the cell protein, but most of the caustics have some subsidiary action which is their own particular characteristic. For instance, silver nitrate reacts with the chlorides of sodium, potassium and other metals in the tissues to form silver chloride. Silver chloride is insoluble and forms a barrier to the further penetration of the silver nitrate into the tissue, so that the silver nitrate has a surface action and actually limits its own penetration. The dark brown-black coagulum is characteristic of the salts of silver which have the property of changing colour on exposure to light. Nitric acid is another caustic which has a surface action. This is due to the fact that it is a powerful oxidizing agent and oxidizes the precipitated protein, thus forming a barrier to its own further penetration. Pyrogallol, on the other hand, has a powerful reducing action. It does not form a barrier and penetrates deeply into the tissues when it is applied in an ointment base. The caustics which are commonly used in chiropody include mono-, di- and tri-chloroacetic acids, silver nitrate, nitric acid, salicylic acid, pyrogallol and potassium hydroxide.

DEODORANTS

A *Deodorant* corrects offensive odours. A medicament which merely masks an odour is not a deodorant.

Deodorants may be used in the condition of bromidrosis where there is excessive sweating with a foul odour, and also for foul ulcerations and septic conditions. Since in cases of bromidrosis it is often sufficient to diminish the flow of sweat the anhidrotics are, *per se*, deodorants. Boric acid is said to act as a deodorant in cases of bromidrosis. It may be used as a saturated solution which is painted on and allowed to dry or as an ingredient of foot powders such as Compound Salicylic Acid Dusting-powder B.P.C. 1963. Flowers of sulphur is also used as an ingredient of deodorant dusting-powders. For foul smelling ulcers and septic conditions an antiseptic having an oxidizing action may be used. These include chlorinated lime and the chlorine antiseptics, "Milton", potassium permanganate, potassium hydroxyquinoline sulphate and sodium perborate. Some of these drugs may be applied also in lotion form to cases of bromidrosis. Mild antiseptics may help by increasing the acidity of the skin when bacterial decay is arrested, e.g. topical amino-acids ("Akileine").

DETERGENTS

A *Detergent* is a substance which has the power, when applied to a solid surface, to remove from it any foreign matter, especially grease.

A detergent acts first of all as a wetting agent. It wets the surface to which it is applied and it also wets the dirt and grease on that surface so that the latter is loosened and adsorbed by the detergent. The detergent causes the formation of an oil-in-water emulsion with the soil from the surface. It is important that this emulsion should be stable and that the soil should remain emulsified until it can be rinsed away. A detergent which deposits the emulsified soil on another part of the surface has no practical value. Some of the dirt on the surface may actually be soluble in the detergent. There are some hundreds of different detergents which are listed and which are used for various purposes. Therefore, only a simplified picture of the group can be presented and only those detergents which may be encountered by the chiropodist are mentioned.

From the section dealing with emulsions it will be seen that a detergent consists of a polar and non-polar end, the polar end being soluble in water and the non-polar end being soluble in oils and fats. Like many other substances when they are dissolved in water, the detergents "ionize", that is to say, the molecule of the detergent splits up into an anion, carrying a negative electrical charge, and a cation, carrying a positive electrical charge. An example of ionization, that of the common salt (which is not a detergent) would be:

$$NaCl \rightarrow Na^+ + Cl^-$$
Cation Anion

The soap $C_{17}H_{33} \cdot COONa$ divides into polar and non-polar ends thus:

Non-polar	Polar
$C_{17}H_{33}$	COONa

but it ionizes thus:

Anion	Cation
$C_{17}H_{33}COO^-$	Na^+

Where the non-polar long carbon chain is the anion the detergent is known as an anionic detergent.

On the other hand, cetrimide divides into polar and non-polar ends thus:

Non-polar	Polar
$C_{16}H_{33}$	$-N-Br$ with $/CH_3$, $\backslash CH_3$, CH_3

and ionizes thus:

Anion	Cation
Br^-	$C_{16}H_{33}(CH_3)N^+$

so that cetrimide has the long carbon chain in the cation and is a cationic detergent.

The detergents may be grouped as:
  (1) Anionic.
  (2) Cationic.
  (3) Non-ionic.

The Anionic Detergents

(a) The soaps. The soaps are the soluble sodium and potassium salts of the long chain fatty acids, e.g.:

$C_{17}H_{33}COOK$ Potassium oleate
$C_{17}H_{33}COONa$ Sodium oleate

The sodium salts give the hard and the potassium salts the soft soaps. Since the calcium and magnesium salts of the fatty acids are not soluble in water, the effectiveness of the soaps is considerably reduced when they are used in hard water, i.e. water containing dissolved calcium and magnesium salts.

(b) The higher fatty alcohols, e.g.:

$C_{12}H_{25}OH$ Lauryl alcohol
$C_{16}H_{33}OH$ Cetyl alcohol
$C_{18}H_{37}OH$ Stearyl alcohol

Cetostearyl alcohol B.P. is an example of this group.

(c) The sulphated fatty alcohols:

$C_{12}H_{25}OSO_3Na$ Sodium lauryl sulphate
                                    ("Sulphonated Lorol")
$C_{16}H_{33}OSO_3Na$ Sodium cetyl sulphate
$C_{16}H_{33}OSO_2Na$ Sodium cetyl sulphonate

These substances are very good wetting agents and detergents, and since their calcium and magnesium salts are soluble they are quite effective in hard water. Sodium Lauryl Sulphate B.P. is an example of this group. Solution of sulphestol ("Teepol") is similar to the sulphonated fatty alcohols. Teepol is used as an auxiliary emulsifying agent, that is to say it is used in conjunction with other emulsifying agents. A 0·5 per cent solution is widely used for cleaning glassware and instruments. It has a marked defatting action.

The Cationic Detergents

The most widely used example of this class of detergent is Cetrimide B.P. which is tetradecyl trimethylammonium bromide. Solution of Benzalkonium Chloride B.P.C. ("Zephiran") and Domiphen Bromide B.P.C. ("Bradosol") are similar quaternary ammonium derivatives.

The cationic detergents have the advantage of being quite strongly germicidal. They are incompatible with the anionic detergents.

The non-Ionic Detergents

These have very little action and are not used topically. This group contains the polymers of high fatty acids using hydrophilic and hydrophobic groups as linkages. The most effective of these are those compounds which have a relatively even distribution of their hydrophilic and hydrophobic groups, e.g. the polyoxyethylene derivatives of fatty acids, e.g. "Polysorbate 65", etc. These detergents are mainly used in washing powders. Other examples of non-ionic detergents are the higher glyceryls although glycerol itself is not a non-ionic detergent. One of the higher glyceryls which is a non-ionic detergent is glyceryl monostearate (Self-emulsifying Monostearin B.P.C.). The polyethylene glycols (Macrogols) fall into this group.

EMOLLIENTS

An *Emollient* is a medicament which softens and lubricates the tissues. The word "soften" is used here in a restricted sense: high strengths of salicylic acid soften the stratum corneum but salicylic acid is not an emollient.

An emollient is generally greasy in nature, the animal fats being preferred to the mineral greases. Emollients maintain the softness of the skin (see p. 117), but at the same time, since they are greasy in nature, they also lubricate the skin and reduce friction between the latter and its surroundings. The use of emollients in chiropody is important in maintaining the good texture and elasticity of the skin. Vegetable oils may also be used as emollients, which generally contain more than one ingredient. The common ingredients include hard and soft paraffin, liquid paraffin, wool fat, wool alcohols, beeswax, olive oil, arachis oil, cod-liver oil and glycerin. Cetyl alcohol is an ingredient of a useful emollient cream, viz.: Cetyl Alcohol 4 per cent, Glycerin 6 per cent, Soft Paraffin 90 per cent. Hydrous Lanolin is a favourite emollient and many ointments act as such by virtue of their bases. Oil-in-water creams and ointments are often useful emollients (see The Semi-solid Preparations, pp. 9–11).

HAEMOSTATICS

A *Haemostatic* is a medicament or other agent which arrests or diminishes haemorrhage. A *Styptic* is a medicament which arrests haemorrhage.

The haemostatics are discussed in Chapter IX, "The Arrest of Haemorrhage".

Examples of haemostatics are:

(*a*) Ferric chloride and silver nitrate which act by precipitating proteins.

(*b*) Calcium alginate which acts by providing a network of fibres which promotes coagulation and then is slowly absorbed by the body. Absorbable gelatin sponge will absorb many times its own weight of blood and permits formation of fibrin plugs at capillary ends. Oxidized cellulose works in the same way but should not be used as a surface dressing except for immediate control of bleeding as it inhibits epithelialization.

(*c*) Adrenaline which exerts a direct action on the blood vessels. Other haemostatics sometimes used in chiropody are ferric subsulphate, alum and copper sulphate.

HEALING AGENTS AND STIMULANTS

A *Healing Agent* is a medicament which promotes healing and healthy granulation. The action of a healing agent is twofold; it has an antiseptic action and it has the power to assist phagocytosis. Probably most of the antiseptics which do not actually interfere with phagocytosis and the formation of healthy granulation tissues may be classed as healing agents. These include the acridines, alcohol, Peru Balsam, Compound Benzoin Tincture, yellow mercuric oxide, cod-liver oil, crystal violet and brilliant green.

In contrast to the healing agents are the stimulants. *Stimulants* are medicaments, such as scarlet red and ichthammol, which stimulate the formation of granulation tissue or those which exert a healing action by stimulating the blood supply and the flow of lymph. The latter are particularly indicated in septic conditions and ulcers which are slow to heal. They include chlorinated lime, Dakin's solution and the chlorine antiseptics, and zinc sulphate.

Like the astringents, the healing agents and stimulants are classified according to their result rather than their action.

Polynoxylin and Clioquinol, "Vioform" (Ciba) have been recently introduced for the treatment of skin and wound infections and for the treatment of ulcerations.

RUBEFACIENTS

A *Rubefacient* is a medicament which, when applied to the skin, produces a mild local inflammation.

The word "counter-irritant" is sometimes used, in chiropody, to mean the same thing as rubefacient. This term, however, refers to the practice of producing inflammation of the skin to relieve pain in some internal organ which is a doubtful way of describing the use of rubefacients in chiropody. A similar result to that produced by the application of a rubefacient may be obtained by the action of heat or of friction on the surface of the skin.

It is interesting to note that many of the rubefacients are used also as fungicides. Rubefacients do not precipitate the protein of cell cytoplasm and, since many of the rubefacients are volatile in nature, they penetrate fairly deeply into the tissues, especially when aided by heat.

Rubefacients which are used in chiropody include camphor, chloral hydrate, iodine, menthol and methyl salicylate. It has already been pointed out that heat acts as a rubefacient.

An excess dose of any of the rubefacients will lead to blistering; rubefacients in the higher strengths which produce blistering are known as *Vesicants*.

SOLVENTS

A *Solvent*, in the restricted sense in which it is frequently used, may be taken to refer to a medicament which dissolves fats and grease and may be used to prepare the skin prior to operating.

The solvents which are used for this purpose in chiropody are alcohol, ether, acetone, carbon tetrachloride, ethyl acetate and, occasionally, benzene and petrol. It is an advantage if a solvent will dissolve rubber adhesive. The solubility of the rubber adhesives used in various brands of strapping and felts seems to vary quite considerably and where one rubber adhesive can be removed quite easily with carbon tetrachloride another brand may be extremely resistant. Ether dissolves most of these adhesives very readily but it has the disadvantages of evaporating so rapidly that the dissolved material may be deposited elsewhere on the skin. After removal of plaster adhesive with ether there is often a vague general stickiness left over the whole of the foot, especially if the adhesive is fairly fresh. Fresh marks left by strapping are better removed with acetone.

Ether is highly inflammable and may form an explosive mixture with oxygen; acetone and alcohol are inflammable; carbon tetrachloride is non-inflammable but its fumes are toxic in quite low concentrations. Ethyl acetate is to be preferred as a general solvent.

CHAPTER III

INFLAMMATION AND REPAIR

"In Nature's battle against disease, the physician is but the helper who furnishes Nature with weapons, the apothecary is but the smith who forges them."—*Paracelsus* (1493–1541)

"We are to admit no more causes of natural things than such as are both true and sufficient to explain their appearances. To this purpose the philosophers say that Nature does nothing in vain when less will serve; for Nature is pleased with simplicity, and affects not the pomp of superfluous causes."—*Newton* (1642–1727)

THROUGH the ages man has regarded life as a struggle against the forces of Nature, a battle in which he is sometimes on the offensive but one in which he is more often defending himself. The "battle against disease" finds man mainly on the defensive and a wise commander, called upon to defend his country, first assesses the natural defences which are at his disposal. Our bodies have ways and means of defending themselves against disease and injury and of overcoming their effects. Before discussing the measures that man can take, the body's own defensive and reparative systems must be examined and understood.

Before embarking on an undertaking it is desirable to know what is its aim. If a group of cells is damaged, the body first sets out to deal with the cause of the damage in order to prevent more injury being done and, second, it replaces with new material the tissues which have been damaged or destroyed. The use of the word "damage" in this context needs some qualification. Take as an example a cut made by a knife in the tissues of the finger. Some immediate damage is done by the knife and this damage is minimized by drawing the finger quickly away from the knife. Other damage is done to the tissue cells by bacteria which enter the cut made by the knife and the body must react to curb such activity and to remove the bacteria. Also, the cells which have been damaged by the knife and by the bacteria must be replaced. The way in which these things are brought about is discussed in the following pages.

"Inflammation" was defined by E. L. Opie in 1910 as "the process whereby cells and exudate accumulate in irritated[1] tissues and tend

[1] Irritated here means damaged or injured. The irritant may be chemical, e.g. an acid; physical, e.g. a cut, sprain or burn; or it may be bacterial, viral, fungal, etc.

to protect them from further injury". This should not be accepted as a complete definition of inflammation but it serves as an idea upon which a wider concept may be based. The exudate mentioned above consists of blood plasma which leaves the capillary blood vessels in copious quantities during the inflammatory process: the cells are the white blood cells and certain other cells which are found in the tissues outside the blood vessels.

The agents in an inflammatory reaction are:

(1) the blood plasma,
(2) the white blood cells,
(3) certain tissue cells.

The whole process of inflammation includes:

(1) the transport of these agents to the irritated tissues,
(2) their activity at the site of irritation,
(3) the removal of the waste products of the reaction.

"Repair" is the reconstruction of the damaged tissues and *it starts almost immediately the damage occurs*. The repair process is synchronous with the inflammatory process and it will be shown that inflammation and repair cannot be regarded as two separate processes but that together they make up the series of events which follows damage to tissue cells.

THE TRANSPORT OF THE CELLS AND EXUDATE TO THE SITE OF IRRITATION

The early stages of inflammation are concerned with the blood vessels and the blood flow which are the means whereby cells and plasma are brought to the site of irritation. The first change in the blood vessels is generally a widening of the minute blood vessels.[1] In some cases this may be preceded by a momentary constriction of the arterioles but this does not always occur. In the skin the vessels which become dilated are those which are normally in use, but in other tissues, such as muscle, kidney and the alimentary tract, there may be an opening-up of vessels which are for most of the time either closed or are open only enough to allow the passage of plasma, but not cells. The immediate dilatation takes place chiefly in the arterioles, less in the veins and least in the capillaries which do not become fully dilated until about an hour after the onset of inflammation.

[1] The minute vessels are the arterioles and venules, together with the capillaries which connect the two former.

When cells are injured they release a chemical material called H-substance[1] which has a double effect:

1. It acts upon certain nerve endings in the dermis and the impulse is conveyed directly to the muscles in the walls of the arterioles. This is unusual since almost all nerve impulses are referred to the central

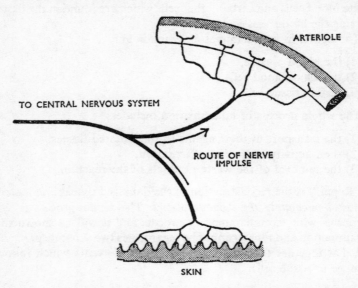

Fig. 7. Diagram of an Axon-reflex: The impulse from the nerve ending in the skin passes along the branch of the afferent nerve to the muscle in the neighbouring arteriole without first travelling to the central nervous system.

nervous system. The direct connection between the receptor organs in the skin and the muscles in the wall of the arterioles is called an axon-reflex. (See diagram.)

2. When sufficient H-substance has collected in the damaged tissues it acts directly on the veins and capillaries causing them to become dilated.

The dilatation of the arterioles by axon-reflex is immediate, but it takes some time for the H-substance to act upon the veins and capillaries.[2]

[1] This chemical substance is very closely allied to histamine, but it has not been proved conclusively that it is identical and it is therefore referred to as H-substance.

[2] For a detailed appreciation of the evidence concerning H-substance and axon-reflex, the reader is referred to the appropriate section in *Applied Physiology* by Samson Wright.

As a result of the dilatation of the minute blood vessels more blood, both cells and plasma, is brought to the irritated area, but the cells and plasma are inside the blood vessels and the damaged cells are on the outside. The next development in the inflammatory reaction is for the cells and plasma to leave the blood vessels.

When the blood vessels first become dilated the rate of flow of blood through the vessels is increased but after some time it falls below the normal rate and in some cases the flow may even cease entirely. The slowing down of the blood stream is thought to be due to loss of fluid from the vessels leading to a marked increase in the viscosity[1] of the blood in the vessels. The loss of fluid is due in the first place to the increased hydrostatic pressure[2] within the capillaries caused by the arteriolar dilatation and later, when the capillaries become dilated, to the increased permeability[3] of the walls of the capillary blood vessels. As the viscosity of the blood increases, the

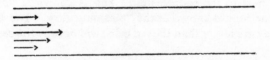

FIG. 8. Diagram of a liquid flowing through a narrow tube: the length of the arrows is proportional to the velocity of the liquid.

greater resistance to flow in the venules raises the hydrostatic pressure in the capillaries so that there is a further loss of fluid and a vicious circle is set up thus:

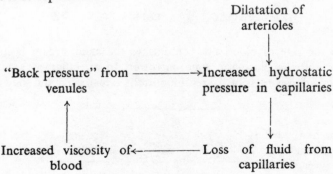

^[1] Viscosity: the tendency to resist flow, e.g. treacle is more viscous than water.

[2] Hydrostatic pressure: here, the outward force exerted by the blood on the vessel walls.

[3] Permeability: allowing the passage of matter. It will be seen from the following pages that there are degrees of permeability.

The white blood cells now leave the vessels and travel to the site of the damaged tissues. When a fluid passes through a narrow tube the velocity of the liquid at the centre of the tube is greater than that at its sides.

If there is a number of particles in the flowing liquid, the largest particles will tend to occupy the more rapidly moving part of the fluid, i.e. the largest particles will occupy the centre of the flow.

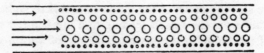

FIG. 9. Diagram showing particles in a liquid flowing through a narrow tube.

When blood is flowing freely through a vessel the cells, red and white, form a moving column at the centre of the tube, leaving a clear zone next to the endothelium.[1] This is known as "axial flow" and the clear zone is known as the "plasmatic flow". The white cells, because they are larger than the red cells, will occupy the centre of the axial flow.

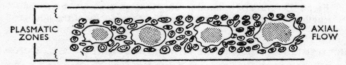

FIG. 10. Blood flowing freely through a vessel (diagrammatic)

White Blood Cells   Red Blood Cells

As the rate of blood flow diminishes the axial stream becomes wider and the plasmatic zone narrower. In an inflamed area the mutual adhesiveness of the red blood cells is increased and they tend

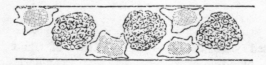

FIG. 11. The margination of the white blood cells.

to clump together. Because the clumps of red cells are now bigger than the individual white cells the clumps of red cells tend to take

[1] Endothelium: the special tissue lining the blood vessels.

the central position and the white cells are pushed towards the margins of the axial flow.

After the white blood cells move to the periphery of the blood stream they begin to adhere to the endothelial lining of the vessels. The white cells are then gradually extruded through small apertures which they make between the endothelial cells and pass through the vessel's walls into the tissue spaces. Usually the gap made by the passage of a white blood cell closes immediately the cell has passed through it, but a few red cells also may be forced through the aperture before it closes.[1]

At the same time as the changes are taking place in the vessels and in the rate of blood flow, exudation of plasma is taking place from the capillary blood vessels. The walls of the capillary blood vessels act as semi-permeable membranes, that is to say, they allow the passage of molecules up to a certain size, including those of water and the dissolved crystalloid[2] molecules but they will not allow the

---

[1] In modern works the forcible extravasation of the red blood cells is referred to as "diapedesis". "Diapedesis", from the Greek, *dia*—through, *pedesis*—leaping, is more generally defined as "the migration of the white blood corpuscles through the walls of the blood vessel without apparent rupture".

[2] If two solutions of different concentrations are separated by a semi-permeable membrane, which will permit the passage of the solvent but not of the dissolved substances, the solvent will tend to flow *from the weak to the strong* concentration and the concentrations tend to become equal. This is called osmosis. Thus:

S.P. MEMBRANE				S.P. MEMBRANE	
		tends to become			2 g. of salt in 133 ml. of water
1 g. of salt in 100 ml. of water	2 g. of salt in 100 ml. of water			1 g. of salt in 66 ml. of water	

The water will tend to flow from the dilute to the concentrated solution.

The osmotic pressure is the force required to prevent the solvent from passing through the semi-permeable membrane. Crystalloids are defined as substances which, in solution, are able to pass through a semi-permeable membrane. This is not altogether a happy definition. Whether a crystalloid such as the salt (sodium chloride) used in the illustration above, will pass through a semi-permeable membrane depends on the permeability of the membrane. Comparison may be made to a similar rather imprecise definition, that of a filter-passing virus. Filters can be made which retain viruses. It is perhaps easier to conceive of crystalloids as being contrasted to colloids, whose molecules are not diffused as separate entities in solution but which group together to form minute aggregates of molecules. Because the molecules of a colloid in solution are clumped together they cannot pass through a semi-permeable membrane which will allow the passage of

passage of the larger colloidal[2] protein molecules. Under normal conditions fluid passes out of a capillary blood vessel at the arterial end and is attracted back into the vessels at the venous end. The force tending to drive the fluid out of the vessel, the filtering force, is the hydrostatic pressure of the blood in the capillaries which is about 32 mm. of mercury at the arterial end and about 12 mm. of mercury at the venous end. The force tending to pull fluid back into the capillaries is an osmotic[2] force, which is due to the fact that the capillary walls are not normally permeable to the protein molecules so that there is greater concentration of these within the vessels than there is outside.

The difference between the osmotic pressure of the fluid inside the vessels and that of the fluid outside the vessels is the net inward force

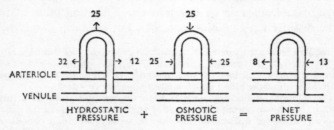

Fig. 12. The pressures in normal capillary blood vessels. The plasma is forced out at the arterial end and is attracted back at the venous end. (All pressures in mm. of mercury.)

of about 25 mm. of mercury attracting fluid back into the vessel. Under normal conditions the outward hydrostatic pressure at the arterial end of the capillary is greater than the inward osmotic

crystalloid molecules. A further difference between crystalloids and colloids is that the former in solution exert a strong osmotic pressure and the latter a small, almost negligible, one.

The theoretical osmotic pressure exerted by the dissolved crystalloids in the blood is the enormous pressure of 6·5 atmospheres or about 4850 mm. of mercury. But this enormous force is cancelled out because the concentration of crystalloids is the same in the tissue fluid as it is in the blood plasma. The colloids in the blood exert an osmotic pressure of about 25 mm. of mercury, but this force is not balanced in the tissue fluids. Thus, under normal conditions, there is:

Blood Plasma		*Tissue Fluid*
Crystalloid Osmotic Pressure	⟵	4850 mm. Hg.
4850 mm. Hg.	⟶	Crystalloid Osmotic Pressure
Colloidal Osmotic Pressure	⟵	25 mm. Hg.
Net Osmotic Pressure	⟵	25 mm. Hg.

pressure so that fluid leaves the vessel; at the venous end the inward osmotic pressure is greater than the outward hydrostatic pressure so that fluid is attracted back into the vessel.

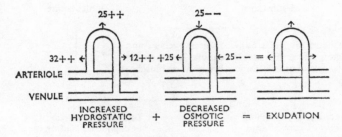

FIG. 13

The exudation in inflammation is due:

(a) to the increased hydrostatic pressure through the whole length of the capillary, and

(b) to the increased permeability of the vessel walls, which allows the large colloidal molecules of globulin and fibrinogen to pass out into the tissue fluid *so that the inward osmotic pressure is decreased.*

The increased permeability of the capillaries was thought to be due to H-substance but recent investigations have demonstrated that it is due to a substance called leucotaxine. Leucotaxine, like H-substance, is due to the partial breakdown of cell protein and is produced when cells are damaged. In addition to the effect of the leucotaxine, it is probable that the stretching of the walls of the capillary blood vessels also increases their permeability.

The diagram on the following page illustrates the means whereby cells and exudate reach the site of irritation.

It will be seen from this diagram that it is the damage done to the tissue cells which initiates the sequel of events bringing the cells and exudate to the irritated tissues and that therefore *the changes are independent of the irritant causing the damage* and are common to all varieties of inflammation.

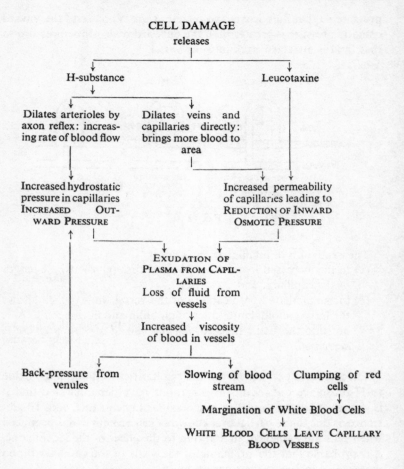

CELL DAMAGE
releases

H-substance — Leucotaxine

Dilates arterioles by axon reflex: increasing rate of blood flow

Dilates veins and capillaries directly: brings more blood to area

Increased hydrostatic pressure in capillaries INCREASED OUTWARD PRESSURE

Increased permeability of capillaries leading to REDUCTION OF INWARD OSMOTIC PRESSURE

EXUDATION OF PLASMA FROM CAPILLARIES
Loss of fluid from vessels

Increased viscosity of blood in vessels

Back-pressure from venules

Slowing of blood stream

Clumping of red cells

Margination of White Blood Cells

WHITE BLOOD CELLS LEAVE CAPILLARY BLOOD VESSELS

THE FUNCTION OF THE CELLS AND EXUDATE AT THE SITE OF IRRITATION

So far, the means whereby the cells and exudate arrive at the site of irritation have been considered. Their function must now be discussed.

The functions of the exudate are:

1. *To dilute bacterial toxins.* Bacteria produce poisons called toxins[1] which damage tissue cells. The ability of the toxins to damage the tissue[2]

---

[1] The question of bacterial toxins is discussed in Chapter IV.
[2] Compare this with the idea that a strong solution of, for example, hydrochloric acid will destroy tissue whereas a dilute solution may not.

depends on their concentration so that the dilution of the toxins renders them less likely to do damage. The dilution of the toxins also lessens the possibility of negative chemotrophism, as will be explained in the following chapter.

2. *To form a barrier round the focus of infection.* The increased permeability of the capillary blood vessels allows the fibrinogen molecules to pass out into the tissue spaces. In the region of the damaged tissues these molecules become converted into fibrin by a mechanism similar to the clotting of blood.[1] The fibrin forms a close meshwork which allows tissue fluid[2] to filter through but which retains particles the size of bacteria. In this way a barrier is formed which tends to localize an infection. The fibrin meshwork also assists the movement of the phagocytes by forming a pavement for their amoeboid movement.

3. *To carry natural antibacterial antibodies to the site of a bacterial infection.* The production of antibodies is specifically initiated by the presence of bacteria.

It will be noticed that all three of the functions of the inflammatory exudate listed above refer, in one way or another, to bacteria, but that exudation occurs whether bacteria are present or not. In this chapter inflammation is dealt with in general terms; the special responses elicited by the presence of bacteria are dealt with separately because it is desirable to establish a clear picture of what happens when tissues are damaged, no matter what causes the injury.

---

[1] *The clotting of blood* may be summarized in simplified form as follows:

(i) The circulating blood contains the soluble protein Fibrinogen and a substance Prothrombin.

(ii) When cells are damaged, an enzyme Thrombokinase is produced, and when blood is shed a factor Thromboplastin is released by the disintegration of certain fragmentary blood cells, the blood platelets, which circulate in normal blood.

(iii) The Thromboplastin and Thrombokinase, in the presence of calcium ions (see page 34) act upon Prothrombin to produce Thrombin.

(iv) The Thrombin converts the soluble Fibrinogen into insoluble Fibrin which forms the blood clot

$$\text{Prothrombin} + \text{Ca}^{++} + \text{Thrombokinase} \rightarrow \text{Thrombin}$$
$$\text{Thrombin} + \text{Fibrinogen} \rightarrow \text{Fibrin}$$

[2] Samson Wright points out: "The lymphatics are a closed system where they ramify in the tissues. A distinction should be drawn between the fluid in the tissue spaces—tissue fluid and that in the lymphatic channels, to which the term lymph should be restricted." I have, therefore, adopted the following nomenclature:

Fluid in the blood vessels	blood plasma
Fluid in the tissue spaces	tissue fluid
Fluid in the lymphatic vessels	lymph

The function of the white blood cells[1] at the site of irritation must next be considered. In the early stages of inflammation it is mainly neutrophil granulocytes, called microphages by Metchnikoff, which leave the vessels and migrate into the irritated tissues. After twelve to twenty-four hours these are followed by the large, slow-moving mononuclear leucocytes or macrophages. The function of the microphages and macrophages is to ingest organic particles such as damaged tissue cells, bacteria, etc., and to digest them by the action of enzymes present in the protoplasm of the microphages and macrophages. This process is known as phagocytosis. The extravasated white blood cells are aided in the process of phagocytosis by other cells called histiocytes, which are present in the tissues outside the blood vessels. The histiocytes are part of the reticulo-endothelial system[2] and normally are inactive. During the inflammatory process they become active and reinforce the work of the microphages and macrophages.

The phagocytes, that is the microphages, macrophages and histiocytes, are capable of amoeboid movement and are attracted towards bacteria and dead cells by a process known as positive chemotrophism. It is the leucotaxine produced by the damaged cells which attracts the phagocytes towards the damaged tissues. Leucotaxine, it will be remembered, also causes increased permeability of the walls of the capillaries. One of the results of the inflammatory products entering the general circulation via the lymphatic system is to cause

[1] The whole class of white blood cells is included in the term leucocytes. There are three main classes of leucocyte:

(1) Granulocytes, which are also called polymorphonuclear leucocytes. Granulocytes are characterized by the presence of granules in the cell protoplasm. According to the way the granules react to staining techniques the granulocytes are divided into Neutrophil Granulocytes (stained by neutral stains), Eosiniphil Granulocytes (stained by acid stains) and Basophil Granulocytes (stained by alkaline or basic stains).

(2) Lymphocytes, which are large round non-granular cells. They are divided into large and small lymphocytes.

(3) Monocytes which form a group of cells which includes the mononuclear, hyaline and transitional cells.

Phagocytes (Greek: eater-cells) are all those leucocytes and other cells which have the property of ingesting particulate foreign bodies including bacteria and dead tissue cells.

Microphage (Greek: little eater) is an alternative name for the granulocyte.

Macrophage (Greek: large eater) is an alternative name for the mononuclear leucocyte.

N.B. The little and large refer to the size of the cell and not to the size of the meal.

[2] The reticulo-endothelial system consists of cells scattered throughout the body having the specialized function of phagocytosis very highly developed. They occur in the spleen, the bone marrow, liver and lymph glands. The histiocytes in the tissues form part of this system.

the liberation of extra granulocytes from the bone marrow, where they are produced, into the blood stream, so that the blood contains an unusually large number of these cells.

PAIN IN INFLAMMATION

In certain diseases the sufferers are incapable of experiencing pain because the incoming sensation never reaches the central nervous system. Such a sufferer may be sitting reading and smoking a cigarette when he suddenly smells burning meat. But it is not the dinner that is ruined. The smell comes from the flesh of his own fingers being burned by the cigarette! The first thing he knows about it is the smell of burning flesh by which time severe damage has been done to the tissues of his fingers—a dramatic story which serves to stress the importance of pain as defence mechanism. The trauma may not be of so violent a nature. In the disease known as tabes, pain sensibility is lost. An injury is inflicted on a joint and a mild sprain or subluxation occurs. Because the patient feels no pain he receives no effective treatment for the inflammation and continues to use the joint so that the condition becomes progressively worse until a very considerable deformity results. Once again, this example shows that pain is an essential defence mechanism.

There is an important law in physiology relating to the impulse carried by a single nerve fibre, called the all-or-none law. This law lays it down that the intensity of impulse set up in any nerve fibre is independent of the strength of the exciting stimulus, provided that the stimulus is adequate. In other words, when a stimulus is applied to an end-organ, the fibre from that organ either does not respond at all or responds to the utmost of its capacity. A simple analogy which is often used to explain the all-or-none law is the firing of a rifle. A certain minimum pressure is required to pull back the trigger, but beyond this minimum pressure any degree of pressure may be applied to the trigger without making the bullet travel any faster. When cells are damaged, yet another substance different from H-substance and leucotaxine, is released. This substance has the effect of making the nerve endings respond more easily to stimuli. To return to the rifle analogy—the minimum force required to pull back the trigger is reduced. The technical expression used to describe this is "lowering of the pain threshold", and the lay term is to say that the part becomes "tender".

Tenderness means that the nerves are sensitive to stimuli to which they would not normally react and a very mild degree of warmth, pressure or friction will cause pain. The slight increase in tension produced by an artery beating nearby produces a throbbing pain. The "pain-substance" released by the damaged cells is stable, that is, it is not easily broken down but persists in the tissues for a long time. It may spread beyond the immediate neighbourhood of the damaged cells and produce a wide area of tenderness.

Tenderness will mean that the part is kept still because it hurts to move it. In the case of infection this will help to keep the infection localized. Tenderness will mean also that the part is used as little as possible, i.e. it is rested. Pain both draws attention to the fact that damage is being done and also serves as a reminder that damage has been done and has not yet been made good.

The outcome of inflammation may be:

1. *Resolution*, when the irritated tissues return to normal without any permanent changes being produced, the products of the inflammatory reaction being absorbed by the lymphatic system.

2. *Organization*, when the tissues concerned are replaced to varying degrees by connective tissue produced as the result of the organization of the inflammatory products.

3. *Destruction of the tissues* (breakdown or necrosis), which is usually followed by repair through granulation, as in healing by second intention.

Of these three, resolution is the most, and destruction the least, desirable outcome.

If the tissues destroyed are those of a free surface, e.g. the skin or a mucous membrane, then an ulcer is formed. Three stages of simple ulceration may be recognized.

1. *Extension*, the period when damage is being done.

2. *A chronic or stationary stage*, when the destruction of the tissues has taken place but when healing has not yet begun, e.g. a broken chilblain. This circumstance will not occur unless there is some factor which interferes with the process of repair. It has been stressed that the repair process is normally synchronous with the inflammatory reaction but, in certain circumstances, for example if there is a defect in the local circulation, venous stasis due to varicose veins, constitutional disorders such as diabetes, pressure due to oedema or continuous irritation, the process of repair may be held up and chronic ulceration may result.

3. *The stage of repair* by granulation.

HEALING PROCESSES

The healing processes may present a less coherent picture than that of inflammation. Much of the work which has been done in recent years has shown that many of the accepted hypotheses concerning healing were, in fact, misconceived. The more recent ideas on the healing of wounds still leave many questions unanswered and have indeed posed new ones, particularly questions relating as to why cells should alter their developmental behaviour and what determines the timing of their alteration in function. Yet the picture presented is a logical one. For instance, damage to the skin results in temporary arrangements to take care of its important functions of defence and homeostasis and a temporary repair fulfils these functions until more permanent arrangements are made. Some stress has been laid on the role of inflammation as a defence mechanism arising from cell damage. Obviously if cells are damaged healing must take place unless the tissue is to die. Therefore repair must commence as soon as damage is done and will take place concomitantly with the inflammatory process. Some text books use the concept that the first part of the healing process is inflammation and this is acceptable. What is important is that repair is not instantaneous and obviously it is necessary for the defensive processes to continue while the damage to the tissue is being made good because, until at least a certain amount of healing has been accomplished, the tissues will not be able to stand up to the normal strains and stresses to which they are subjected.

Distinction may usefully be drawn between the terms "healing", "repair" and "regeneration". "Healing" implies the re-establishment of tissue continuity such as may follow any injury and includes both regeneration and repair. "Regeneration" implies the reconstruction of the original architecture of any organ or tissue in response either to wear and tear or to superficial abrasions or damage. The epidermis is particularly notable for its powers of regeneration. "Repair" implies that a wound heals but without the restoration of the original architecture of the tissue but with varying degrees of usually permanent distortion or architectural disorganisation. A substantial "full-thickness" injury to the skin, that is where there is involvement of both dermis and epidermis as well as the subcutaneous tissue, may result in the architecture of the skin being changed to a greater or lesser extent by the formation of scar tissue which is the repair material of the skin. In this case the repair material is closely allied

THE EVENTS FOLLOWING CELL DAMAGE

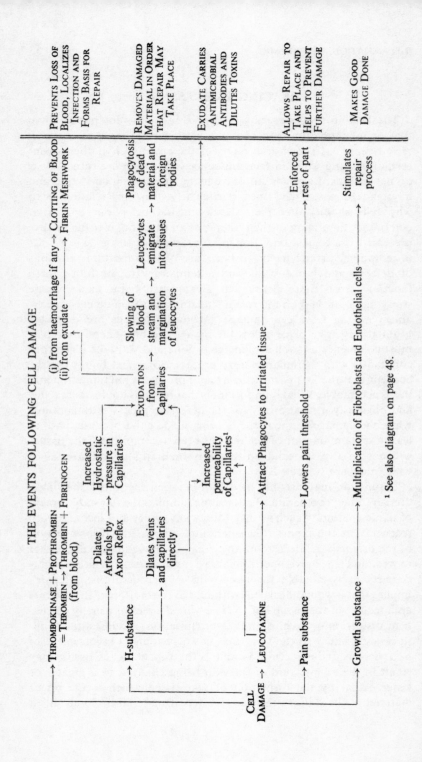

CELL DAMAGE →

→ THROMBOKINASE + PROTHROMBIN = THROMBIN + FIBRINOGEN (from blood) → (i) from haemorrhage if any → CLOTTING OF BLOOD (ii) from exudate → FIBRIN MESHWORK — PREVENTS LOSS OF BLOOD, LOCALIZES INFECTION AND FORMS BASIS FOR REPAIR

→ H-substance → Dilates Arteriols by Axon Reflex → Increased Hydrostatic pressure in Capillaries → EXUDATION FROM CAPILLARIES

Dilates veins and capillaries directly → Increased permeability of Capillaries[1]

→ Slowing of blood stream and margination of leucocytes → Leucocytes emigrate into tissues → Phagocytosis of dead material and foreign bodies — REMOVES DAMAGED MATERIAL IN ORDER THAT REPAIR MAY TAKE PLACE

EXUDATE CARRIES ANTIMICROBIAL ANTIBODIES AND DILUTES TOXINS

→ LEUCOTAXINE → Attract Phagocytes to irritated tissue

→ Pain substance → Lowers pain threshold → Enforced rest of part — ALLOWS REPAIR TO TAKE PLACE AND HELPS TO PREVENT FURTHER DAMAGE

→ Growth substance → Multiplication of Fibroblasts and Endothelial cells → Stimulates repair process — MAKES GOOD DAMAGE DONE

[1] See also diagram on page 48.

to the normal tissue but there is a greater amount of collagen and the repair site does not fulfil normal skin functions.

Most superficial lesions of the skin heal by true regeneration. This is manifestly so since the average skin is relatively unscarred in spite of the many minor traumata to which it is subjected. However, many cutaneous wounds heal by repair with the formation of scar tissue. Even in the case of the skin alone several types of healing may be described, for example the "healing" of a partial thickness skin-graft or a graze; healing by primary intention where the continuity of the tissue is disrupted but there is no loss of tissue; or healing of a wound by secondary intention where there has been actual loss of tissue. It is the last two types of healing which are of greatest concern to the chiropodist.

The general sequence of events is as follows. The blood in the wound clots in the manner described on page 49. This is a "logical" step to prevent loss of blood and the fibrin meshwork laid down forms a tenuous sort of repair. The surface of the blood clot becomes dehydrated and forms the familiar scab which is nature's dressing. The scab temporarily takes over the functions of the lost epidermis in preventing water vapour loss and in giving protection against bacteria and the entry of foreign bodies. The scab is formed by the serous exudate losing water to the air and at about the end of the first day a balance is reached where the loss of water from the surface is balanced by rewetting of the tissue from below. This point of of balance is below the wound surface and is in the dermis, so that a thin layer of dermal tissue is incorporated with the serous fluid in the scab. The dried layer of the dermis is too dehydrated to support cell life so that the accumulation of leucocytes, which is a feature of the inflammatory process following cell damage, means that the leucocytic layer forms in the dried tissue underneath. The naturally formed scab is continuous with the viable fibrous tissue and there is no layer of separation. The scab is eventually detached by proteolytic enzymes released by the regenerating epidermis growing beneath it.

The first tissue to regenerate is the epidermis and no connective tissue regeneration takes place until a new epithelial layer has been established. The new epidermis is produced directly from the existing epidermis at the edge of the wound and also from the remains of any epidermal appendages which may have been left in the wound—hair follicles, sebaceous glands and sweat ducts. Each of these sources of epidermis responds with a burst of mitotic activity reaching a peak on the third day of as much as twenty times the normal rate. The epidermal cells move actively across the wound surface as a sheet of tissue underneath the scab. Exactly how they move is not known but it is likely that the tissue rolls over with a "leap frog" progress of cells.

The mitotic burst is controlled by one of a family of chemical messengers called chalones which have been likened to hormones except in so far as they inhibit activity rather than stimulate it. Chalones are produced by the mature cells of the tissue concerned and are specific to that type of tissue only. If the amount of chalone in the fluid bathing the cells falls below a certain critical level then the inhibition is removed and the cells mitose. When sufficient mature cells have been produced the chalone level rises, mitosis is inhibited and in the case of the skin, the cells become keratinocytes rather than mitotic cells. Chalone trips the switch which selects for mitosis or for function.

After the epidermis has grown across the surface of the wound, changes begin to take place in the dermal tissues which have hitherto remained comparatively inactive. It must be noted that the blood clot as such plays no direct part in the repair process and indeed may retard healing until the macrophages have removed the extravasated blood. The order of events in the healing of an incised wound has been summarised thus. During the first two days there is a non-proliferative inflammation corresponding to the exudative stage with vasodilation, oedema and accumulation of neutrophil phagocytic cells. During the second and third days the mononuclear blood cells, tissue histiocytes and/or fibroblasts continue the phagocytic processes. New blood vessels grow into the coagulum. These originate from the injured vessels in the adjacent dermis. The tissue becomes highly vascularised and is known as granulation tissue.

The fibrocytes resident in the dermis play no part as such in its repair. It is now thought that new fibroblasts originate from mononuclear cells some of which are present in the tissue and some of which arrive as the result of the inflammatory process. These enter the exudate and there multiply by mitosis and thereafter synthesise fibroblasts. This is followed by the formation of the components of the dermal ground substance, collagen and eventually fibrous tissue.

At first the new connective tissue forming the sub-epidermal exudate is mostly cellular in its composition: reticulin and collagen fibres do not appear until about the tenth day after the initial wounding. Once the connective tissue has been formed between the new surface epithelial sheet and the denuded dermal tissues the overlying epithelium thickens considerably and sends down rete-peg-like projections into the new connective tissue. In time these projections are absorbed and leave a straight scar-like dermo-epidermal junction. New collagen fibres are formed by the new cellular connective tissue. Surprisingly, the newly formed collagen and reticulin fibrils are not at first aligned, as might be expected in the case of an incised wound, across the incision but lie along the plane of incision at right angles to the surface of the wound. Only after some seven or eight days do the fibrils start to be aligned to the skin surface. As time passes the bundles of collagen become thicker and more densely packed and are aligned along the lines of tension in the scar. The metabolic demands of the scar tissue being low the blood vessels are absorbed into adjacent blood vessels and the scar tissue becomes relatively avascular. Further contraction of the collagenous repair may cause the scar to become puckered. The timetable of healing depends in part on the nature of the wound whether it be a graze, split-skin graft, incision or full-thickness loss wound. In incisions the epithelium crosses the wound in twenty-four hours, it takes longer in full-thickness losses but even where considerable amounts of skin have been lost a tenuous epithelial covering is acquired in five to seven days. Wounds will not heal in the absence of vitamin C and wound healing may be delayed by systemic disease or local micro-angiopathies and peripheral neuropathies.

DEGREES OF INFLAMMATION

So far, a general picture has been given of the way in which the body avoids injury to its tissues and the way in which it makes good damage done to certain types of tissue. The two great standbys of any discussion on inflammation, the classical signs, *rubor, calor, dolor et tumor*,[1] and the division of inflammation into acute and chronic inflammation, have not so far been mentioned. The former are merely the signs by which the state of inflammation may be recognized: the redness and heat being due to the extra blood in the area: pain being caused by the tenderness resulting from the inflammatory reaction and the swelling by the formation of the exudate. In certain stages of inflammation some of the signs may be absent.

The distinction between "acute" and "chronic" inflammation is worthy of detailed discussion. First the meaning of the words should be considered. According to the Oxford English Dictionary, "acute", in the relevant sense, means "coming to a crisis": and "chronic" means "lingering, lasting or inveterate". It is interesting that the Concise Oxford Dictionary records the use, or rather the misuse,

[1] *Rubor, Calor, Dolor et Tumor* (Latin) redness, heat, pain and swelling.

of the word "chronic" in the sense of "bad, intense or severe". "Chronic", from the Greek word *khronos* meaning time,[1] *refers to duration and not to degree.* This gives a useful starting point for discussion.

We have considered several things which happen when cells are damaged. This damage[2] may occur:

1. *As the result of a single event,* e.g. a sprain, a clean cut, a burn. The whole of the damage is done at the outset and the sequence of events which follows cell destruction will be uninterrupted provided that the general condition of the body is satisfactory.

2. *As the result of repeated irritation,* e.g. a toe stubbing against the end of a shoe, repeated trauma of the tissues over a metatarsal head due to an anatomical defect, etc. All the damage does not occur at once, indeed the damage following any single event may be very slight indeed. Following the first injury the inflammatory and repair processes are set in motion but while they are taking place, fresh damage is done to the tissues. One of two things may then occur, a fresh inflammatory and reparative process may start in the normal way, or the tissues may be, as it were, so busy dealing with the first injury that either they cannot respond efficiently to the subsequent injury or they may not be able to deal with it at all. If, for instance, the inflamed tissues have reached a stage when the flow in the blood vessels has slowed down, they cannot respond with an increase in the rate of blood flow at one and the same time. Of course it is not always the same cells which are injured but even a' mild inflammatory response extends beyond the immediate locality of the damaged cells.

In tissues which are being repeatedly injured there may be found, co-existing, all stages of the inflammatory process and all stages of the repair process. If the net rate of cell damage is greater than the rate at which the damaged cells are replaced, the total number of unreplaced damaged cells will increase and necrosis, or death of the tissues, may occur. If the defence and repair mechanisms are more effective than the irritant, the number of damaged cells which have not been replaced will remain fairly constant but there will always be some unreplaced damaged cells for as long as the irritation continues and the inflammation will last over a long period of time, i.e. the inflammation will be chronic. The inflammatory and repair processes may also be prolonged if, for any reason, the tissues cannot respond

---

[1] Cf.: *Chrono*meter, syn*chron*ous, ana*chron*ism, etc.
[2] Damage by bacteria is omitted for the time being and will be considered in a later chapter,

with the series of changes which cell damage evokes. The most common cause of a chronic inflammation of this nature is a deficiency in the circulation of the blood.

Chronic inflammation differs from acute inflammation in the length of time during which the inflammation lasts. At this point, the *enfant terrible* of a class may ask how long an inflammation must last before it can be regarded as being chronic. The answer to this question is to ask for the definition of a moustache. Does one hair on the upper lip constitute a moustache? Do two? Do three, four ... twenty? Obviously, a couple of hundred hairs on the upper lip would constitute a moustache of sorts, but where exactly does the division between moustache and non-moustache lie? This is a common trick of argument and, in fact, acute and chronic inflammation cannot be defined in terms of time alone.

The important point to grasp is this, the changes which occur in inflammation and repair, as these have been discussed so far, are initiated by one thing—damage to tissue cells. If the damage is the result of a single event the changes will occur in uninterrupted sequence provided that the body is in good health. This may be called acute inflammation. If the irritant causes a repetitive series of injury or if the irritant is prolonged in its action, all stages of the inflammatory process and all stages of the repair process may be found going on at the same time. This may be called chronic inflammation. Acute inflammation may be likened to a choir singing in unison or in harmony: chronic inflammation to the same choir singing a round or catch:

1st Voice: London's Burning!! Look yonder!! Fire!!! Fire!!! Bring water! etc.

2nd Voice: Bring water! London's Burning!! Look yonder!! Fire!!! Fire!!! etc.

3rd Voice: Fire!!! Fire!!! Bring water!! London's burning! Look yonder!!! etc.

4th Voice: Look yonder!! Fire!!! Fire!!! Bring water!! London's burning! etc.

Acute inflammation may be mild or severe according to the amount of damage done. Chronic inflammation may likewise be mild or severe according to the net number of damaged cells existing at any one time. Acute inflammation generally comes to a crisis and produces a definite result within a period of time: either the inflammation is successful or death of tissue will occur. Chronic inflammation may also come to a crisis which will produce a definite result as, for example, in the case of a traumatic bursitis. This, generally, is not the result of a single major trauma but of repeated minor traumata. At first the inflammation is quite mild but the irritation continues and the tissues are unable to respond with the normal defence mechanism so that a greater amount of damage will be done by the

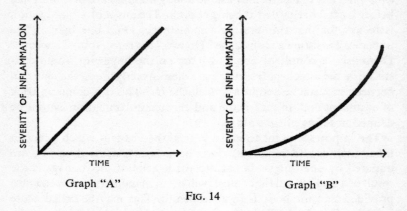

Graph "A"   Graph "B"

FIG. 14

equivalent stimulus. The inflammation increases in severity not at a steady rate as in Graph A, but with a gathering speed as in Graph B.

In course of time the accumulation of the products of cell damage becomes such that the tissues over a wide area respond with an intense inflammatory reaction which may lead to the restoration of normal conditions or, if much tissue has been destroyed, to healing by granulation. In chronic inflammation the pain will become increasingly intense owing to the accumulation of pain-substance in the tissues and while, in the early stages, the pain may cause little inconvenience, as the inflammation becomes more severe the pain will become such that attention is drawn sharply to the fact that something is wrong, and the part will be immobilized and rested.

To sum up, chronic inflammation differs from acute inflammation mainly in that:

1. In acute inflammation there is a fairly straightforward series of events due to a single injury.

2. In chronic inflammation all stages of the inflammatory and repair processes are found synchronously because the irritation persists over a long period. Chronic inflammation may also occur where the normal response of the tissues to injury is impaired in any way.

CHAPTER IV

DEFENCE AGAINST MICROBIAL
INFECTION

INFLAMMATORY reaction, so far, has been discussed in general terms as being the sequence of events following cell damage. When the cause of the damage is the activity of micro-organisms, especially bacteria and viruses, special defence reactions take place which deal both with the living organisms responsible for this activity and their toxins. This chapter deals with the various defence mechanisms of the body which are brought into play when cell damage is caused by infection with micro-organisms. When the response to cell damage was discussed, it was stressed that the events which take place are common to all forms of cell damage. In contrast, many of the defences against microbial infection are often highly specific, and are mobilized only when microbes are present and are effective *only against the organisms initiating them.* These basic defence mechanisms are interdependent and highly complex systems which can be arbitrarily divided into the following sections.

HUMORAL AND CHEMICAL DEFENCES

In most cases of bacterial infection it is the poison, or toxin, produced which damages the tissue cells. Bacterial toxins are of two kinds, exotoxins and endotoxins. Exotoxins are produced by living bacteria and diffuse from the bacterial cells into the medium in which the cells are growing. Probably the best known example of an exotoxin-producing bacterium is *Corynebacterium diphtheriae.* In diphtheria, colonies of bacteria, situated generally in the throat, produce toxins which diffuse and cause harmful effects all over the body. Other bacteria which produce exotoxins are those responsible for gas gangrene, tetanus and scarlet fever. These latter bacteria depend to a great degree on exotoxins for their high virulence and systemic effects. In the majority of pathogens, particularly those affecting the lower limb, it is a combination of their toxins and the allergic phenomenon which determine their pathogenicity. Endotoxins are substances in the cell walls of bacteria which are liberated only in a soluble form after the partial decomposition of the cells. *Pseudo-*

61

monas pyocyanea, a common wound contaminent is an example of
an endotoxin-producing bacterium. Endotoxins are not nearly as
powerful as exotoxins and rely for their effect on gaining high concentrations in the tissues following the death of bacteria. When tissues
are subjected to bacterial infection, substances called antibodies
are produced in the reticulo-endothelial system. Antibodies are
serum proteins produced in response to the presence of an antigen
in the body fluids. An antibody will react specifically to the presence
of a particular organism or toxin and its production is initiated by
the organism or toxin concerned. Once an infection has cleared away
very frequently some antibodies remain ready to deal with future
infection by the same or similar organisms. The mechanism of
antibody production is very complicated and is beyond the scope
of this present work. The reader is referred to the chapters dealing
with immunity in the standard text-books on bacteriology. Antibodies are plasma proteins called immunoglobulins which react with
an antigen. An antibody is specific in that it will only react with the
antigen which has initiated its appearance. An antigen is usually a
foreign protein or occasionally a polysaccharide which may be a
component of a bacterial cell wall or viral particle. This antigen is
usually but not always a pathogenic or toxic substance.

Antibodies have been classified according to their behaviour or
the effects that they exhibit.

1. *Agglutinins.* These antibodies cause the bacterial cells to clump
together or agglutinate which enhances the process of phagocytosis.

2. *Precipitins.* These antibodies cause the precipitation of soluble
antigen on the surface of the invading micro-organism which is then
dealt with readily by phagocytic cells.

3. *Opsonins.* These are very important antibodies. They prepare
or sensitize bacterial cells or other foreign protein matter so that they
become susceptible to phagocytosis. Phagocytosis of certain bacteria
and other particles cannot take place until they have been coated with
a layer of the antibody.

4. *Antitoxins.* When the antigenic determinant is a toxin as with
tetanus or diptheria, the antibody which neutralises it is called an
antitoxin.

Other nomenclature derived from the chemical structure of antibodies is now in more general use. Blood serum contains two principal
groups of plasma proteins, albumins and globulins. The globulins
have been found to be of three fractions, alpha, beta and gamma.
Antibodies are found chiefly among the gammaglobulins. Of these
gammaglobulins, or immunoglobulins, three major and two minor

forms of antibodies have been identified. These five types are labelled G, M, A, D, E, and are given the prefix "Ig" meaning immunoglobulin.

1. IgG—the largest group of antibodies constituting 85 per cent of all antibodies. When infection occurs these are not the first to appear. They are those which tend to give life-long immunity to certain diseases such as measles and chicken pox.

2. IgM—These are the first type of antibody to be produced by the body in response to infection but in most cases are later replaced by the IgG type.

3. IgA—These are much less common than IgG and IgM. They are associated with mucous membranes and tend to give resistance to respiratory tract infections and the like. It has been found that hospital populations are ten times more likely to be deficient in this antibody group when compared with the normal population.

4. IgD—Small quantites of these antibodies are found in the blood but their exact purpose is unknown.

5. IgE—This group of antibodies is associated with immediate hypersensitivity reactions.

There are in the tissues and body fluids other chemical substances which are non-specific in that they will defend the body against any invading organisms.

1. *Complement* is a complex substance consisting of nine or more components. This participates in and greatly enhances (a) cell membrane lysis, (b) phagocytosis, (c) intracellular digestion, (d) chemotaxis, and (e) the immune adherence of bacteria to body cells.

2. *Interferon* is a group of non-specific antiviral agents which are liberated from a cell when it becomes infected by a virus. It may also be stimulated by and active against a wide range of rickettsiae, protozoa and bacteria. The presence of this substance prevents the micro-organism from utilizing the materials of other cells for reproduction. This characteristic of interferon may well be an explanation of the phenomenon of "viral interference" whereby a host, or certain tissue of a host, is able to resist concomitant viral infection. This is because, unlike antibodies, interferon may act against many organisms, not just the specific agent which has initiated its production.

3. *Lysozyme* is a ubiquitous substance which is active against certain pathogens, for example, strains of *Staphylococci* and *Streptococci*.

4. *Lactic acid* is found in sweat and is active against some *Streptococci* and *Escherichia coli*. Lactic acid is also an intermediary metabolite in the tissues at the site of septic inflammation and exerts

a bactericidal effect. In cases of local tissue infection in diabetic patients, the increased acidity is not due to lactic acid but to other non-bactericidal acids.

The part played by the cells in a microbial inflammation must next be considered.

CELLULAR DEFENCES

Phagocytes are of two basic types:
(1) Microphages or polymophonuclear leucocytes.
(2) Macrophages.

The polymorphs (white blood cells) are produced in the bone marrow and released into the blood stream. When infection occurs the number produced increases considerably. The "white cell count" is often used to determine the presence of and sometimes the nature of an in-infection. The macrophages are free cells, called histiocytes, when they occur in the body tissues and monocytes when in the blood. These white cells are all capable of amoeboid movement. There are also fixed macrophages (reticulo-endothelial cells) in the lymph nodes and else-where. The phagocytes are attracted towards the bacteria and to a lesser extent towards damaged leucocytes and tissue cells by a process known as positive chemotrophism. The chemotrophic response depends on the agent eliciting that response. The pyococci (*Staphylococci*, *Streptococci* and other pus-producing organisms) elicit a powerful chemotrophic response while the tubercle bacillus and the typhoid bacillus elicit only a poor chemotrophic response in the neutrophil granulocytes. The agent which elicits the chemotrophic response is a polypeptide which has been given the name leucotaxine. This substance also increases capilliary permeability. Certain very virulent bacteria elicit a negative chemotrophic response, that is they repel the leucocytes instead of attracting them. It is probable that this property is, in itself, part of the reason for their virulence. In a mixed infection caused by more than one type of bacterium, the phagocytes are preferably attracted towards the less virulent bacteria, that is to say they will attack the less virulent organisms rather than the more virulent types. Other bacteria are capable of being ingested by phagocytes without being killed. They are then protected from humoral defences and may possibly set up a subsequent infection when the phagocyte dies. It has already been mentioned that one of the important fuctions of the inflammatory exudate is to prepare bacteria and other foreign particles for phagocytosis by coating them with opsonins. It is interesting that phagocytes ingest bacteria far more successfully if they can "corner" them against some obstruction in the tissues such as another cell or perhaps the fibrin meshwork laid down by the inflammatory exudate, a process called "surface phagocytosis". Alternatively a number of phagocytes may surround a bacterium in order that one of their number may ingest it. In cases of tuberculosis the phagocytes may unite together to form large multi-nuclear cells sharing a common protoplasm.

In the early stages of an infection, many of the polymorphs ingest bacteria and die. This disintegration of polymorphs and microbes leads to the formation of pus. Later in the infection macrophages predominate and ingest bacteria, dead polymorphs and tissue debris. However, much of the exudate from the inflammatory process is removed from the tissues via the lymphatic system. The minute lymphatic capillaries unite in order to form larger vessels in much the same way as the venules unite to form veins. The lymphatic system is so arranged that no lymph is returned to the main blood stream without first having passed through at least one lymph node. The lymph nodes act as filters and the lymph percolates past a succession of reticulo-endothelial cells with highly developed powers of phagocytosis which remove from the lymph all particulate matter including bacteria. If viable organisms enter the lymphatic vessels they cause an inflammatory reaction or lymphangitis. When the lymph nodes themselves become infected this is called lymphadenitis. Bacteraemia or septicaemia will ensue if the progress of the infection is not halted at the lymph glands. Two points with regard to the filtration of lymph by the lymph nodes are of practical importance. First, if they are subjected to a prolonged or continuous strain, the nodes are apt to become fatigued and to allow the passage of some particles. Second, the efficiency of filtration is improved if the flow rate of incoming lymph is diminished. Lymph is squeezed along the vessels by the action of the surrounding muscles; hence the importance of rest and immobilization in the management of cases of acute inflammation due to bacterial infection.

ANATOMICAL BARRIERS

The epithelial coverings and linings of the body surfaces, the skin in particular, provide an effective barrier to micro-organisms preventing their penetration to the body tissues. Whereas the body surfaces have many bacteria, both resident commensals and transient organisms (an estimated 60,000 per square inch), the subcutaneous tissues are sterile. On the skin surface "non-pathogenic" bacteria exist in this environment as commensals and although not one of the body's innate defences, these commensals have a strong inhibitory effect on many virulent pathogenic invaders. They may: (1) use all the existing nutrient available on the skin, so preventing the establishment of a strong foothold of pathogens, or (2) provide the wrong chemical environment for pathogens. Other commensals, e.g. diphtheroids and some species of *Staphylococci*, may actually produce antibiotic substances to inhibit other bacteria. The balance, however, between commensalism and pathogenicity is a delicate one and wounds, particularly on the lower limb, may become secondarily infected by these otherwise non-pathogenic bacteria which then inhibit healing. Commensals commonly found in such wounds include, for example, *Streptococcus faecalis or Staphylococcus albus*. These resident micro-organisms, which constitute the normal bacterial flora of the skin are extremely resistant to scrubbing with soap and water and to skin disinfection. They can never be completely removed. Nearly all bacteria can break through the epithelial barrier only when its continuity has been broken by wounds. There are many pathogenic organisms which live on the surface of the skin but which cannot penetrate the skin unless an entrance is made for them.

The most important method by which the skin rids itself of microbes is by desquamation. As squames are shed from the upper layers of the skin so too are the micro-organisms. Bacilli do not survive drying out on these epidermal rafts but most cocci maintain their pathogenicity for remarkably long periods. Acidity of the skin due to fatty acids of its secretions is bactericidal for some *Streptococci* and *Pseudomonas pyocyanea*. The "acid-mantle" of the skin is an important mechanism whereby the skin rids itself of bacteria and fungi or inhibits their growth on the skin surface. Mycotic infections will occur far more frequently on the skin when its normal chemistry is upset. Once pathogens have penetrated to the subcutaneous tissues, the deeper anatomical structures, such as fascias, which divide the deeper tissues into compartments, serve to localize and stop the spread of an infection. New barriers may also be formed by the inflammatory process in the form of fibrin walls laid down around an abscess.

FACTORS MODIFYING RESISTANCE

The tissues of the feet are particularly prone to bacterial, mycotic and wart virus infections due to the effects of minor trauma and their relatively unclean environment. The effects of general debility due to systemic disorders and constitutional factors must also be considered. It is common for one to refer to a person as being "sickly", as catching any illness prevalent at the time. These are, of course, subjective observations and may be totally unjustified, but what are the factors which will make one individual or one race of people, or children rather than adults, "catch" something? The racial, familial or even individual genetic characteristics may obviously affect the resistance to certain micro-organisms. Many viral infections in Europe, e.g. measles, have fatal consequences to comparatively isolated races of South America. Europeans have been exposed for many thousands of years to certain microbes whereas other races have only been exposed for a short time. The age and sex of individuals plays a part in determining susceptibility to certain diseases. Children tend to be susceptible to bacterial infections but relatively resistant to viral diseases, whereas the converse is generally true for adults. Young women are more susceptible to tuberculosis than young men but the situation is reversed in middle age. Other factors such as nutritional deficiencies, social conditions, temperature and climate will alter individual resistance to microbial infection.

Particularly in the lower limb, an impairment in the peripheral circulation leads to a lowering of resistance to infection by diminishing the inflammatory response. Diabetes melitus, the metabolic disorder characterized by deficiency in the hormone insulin, may be responsible for diminished resistance to infection either directly by the upset in tissue metabolism, or indirectly by its long-term deleterious effects on the peripheral vascular and nervous systems.

Corticosteroids are now widely used to suppress the clinical manifestations in diseases such as rheumatoid arthritis, acute rheumatic fever, allergic disorders and inflammatory skin conditions. They are also used for a number of other systemic diseases. In a later chapter when the treatment of aseptic inflammation is discussed, it will be seen that, during treatment, certain aspects of the inflammatory process are suppressed locally by physical means or the local application of medicaments. The anti-inflammatory action of the corticosteroids is far more fundamental and suppresses the biochemical mechanisms which produce the inflammatory response. Inflammation has been presented as a defence mechanism and it is clear that if the inflammatory process is suppressed by the systemic use of corticosteroids the patient is at risk both to infection and to the effects of trauma. The resistance of the patient is lowered. The topical use of corticosteroids has the same effects locally.

The effects of the corticosteroids are extremely complex and the following account of their action is greatly simplified. The lymphocytes contain gamma globulin within their cytoplasm and are of considerable importance in determining the level of antibodies in the blood. It is variously held that they are producers or carriers of antibodies. The release of antibodies from the lymphocytes is under the direct control of the adrenal cortex through the mediation of the hormone cortisone, which in turn is subject to pituitary control through the mediation of ACTH. It has been shown that following injection of either of these hormones the lymphocyte count in the blood falls by up to one half. The rapid disintegration of the lymphocytes liberates large amounts of gamma globulin into the blood stream, which probably accounts for the value of these hormones in the treatment of asthma and allied allergic manifestations. Other effects of these steroids are, however, likely to be deleterious, especially in the presence of virulent infections. They cause a marked depression in the vascular response in inflammation. Phagocytic activity is reduced: the polymorphonuclear leucocytes are directly affected both in number and, more importantly, in their activity. The number of macrophages in the circulation is reduced and the margination of the leucocytes is affected so that the process of diapedesis also suffers. Repair processes are also impaired and it has been shown that the growth of granulation tissue is inhibited.

With the administration of corticosteroids, resistance to infection is lowered, latent infections may be roused to activity and exacerbation of chronic infections is likely. However, the benefits derived from their proper use outweigh the disadvantages. In prescribing or carrying out treatments of patients who are being treated with corticosteroids their effects on resistance of infection and on the inflammatory and repair processes must always be taken into account. It is important that the chiropodist should know whether the patient is receiving such treatment. Most patients receiving this treatment will have been warned about the side-effects and will tell the chiropodist that they are being treated with corticosteroids. This does not free the chiropodist from the responsibility of finding out for himself whether a patient is receiving such treatment. It is just as important to know whether patients are receiving corticosteroid therapy as it is to know whether they are diabetic.

CHAPTER V

PRE-OPERATIVE PROCEDURE

IN the last chapter the natural defences of the body against bacterial infection were considered. The next two chapters deal with the steps which are taken to prevent the entry of bacteria into a wound or abrasion, and so causing infection. These steps are sometimes referred to as *aseptic technique* or *asepsis*, in contrast to the methods used to remove or control bacteria which have entered a wound and which are referred to as *antiseptic technique* or *antisepsis*. In order to minimize the chances of air-borne infection the operator should work in surroundings which are reasonably clean and free from dust. The skin of the operator's hands and of the patient's feet should be free, as far as is possible, from pathogenic micro-organisms: and the knives and other instruments which are used on the feet must be sterilized. The skin cannot be sterilized without serious damage being done to the tissues: it is not possible to remove from it all micro-organisms, pathogenic and non-pathogenic, without destroying the tissues.

There are two groups of bacteria found on the skin—the non-residents (or transient population) which are acquired mainly by contact; and the resident population, which is permanent. The transient bacterial population is loosely attached to the skin by grease and fats and is of course most abundant where the skin is exposed and has the opportunity of being so invaded. It is also very abundant under the free edge of the nails and in such sites as the nail sulci, between the toes, etc. It consists of both pathogenic and non-pathogenic bacteria. This group of bacteria is fairly easily removed by careful scrubbing with a nail brush and soap and water, or by means of detergents, or grease- and fat-solvents. An important point is that the removal of this transient population depends largely on the vigour with which the scrubbing or swabbing is carried out. There is no doubt that a swab of cotton wool which is held in the fingers can be used more effectively than one held in forceps.

The resident population is not easily removed by mechanical means but it is, fortunately, mainly non-pathogenic. Pathogenic organisms may become resident if the skin is exposed to them for long periods. Such organisms as *Staphylococcus aureus, Escherichia*

69

coli and *Pseudomonas pyocyanea* may become resident in this way. It is important, therefore, to remove from the skin without delay any pathogenic contamination, such as that surrounding a septic lesion, otherwise re-infection may occur.

The skin tends to rid itself of micro-organisms by desquamation of the surface cells, and by desiccation, that is depriving bacteria of all moisture. The acidity of the skin due to the fatty acids of the sweat is also a most important factor which enables the skin to rid itself of micro-organisms and this must be borne in mind when using detergents on the skin. The over-enthusiastic use of detergents may remove these fatty acids from the skin and leave it without one of its main forms of protection. It is a matter of common sense that if the skin is dirty there will be a very large transient population of bacteria and that it will have many more organisms to deal with than it is capable of destroying. Hence the aesthetic cleanliness of the skin, particularly that of the feet, is of great importance.

There are two things to be considered in the pre-operative cleansing —the operator's hands and the patient's feet.

The method of preparation for the operator's hands which is almost universally adopted is scrubbing with a nail brush and soap and water. Particular attention must be paid to the cleanliness of the nails. This method serves to eliminate most of the pathogenic bacteria since nearly all the transient population will be removed and there are few pathogenic bacteria among the resident population on the skin. Because the hands are being scrubbed frequently during the day's work, there is little chance for a large resident population to be acquired. This method does not lead to the de-fatting of the operator's skin as the use of a more powerful detergent than soap and water might do. The use of preparations such as Steriloderm and pHisoHex as a routine application after washing the hands, builds up a protective film on the skin which affords a good measure of protection to the operator.

The skin of the patient's feet may be prepared by various methods. It may be prepared by applying an antiseptic to the skin in order to destroy the micro-organisms; alternatively, a detergent or a solvent may be used to remove from it the fat and grease and, with them, the transient bacterial population. There are two important considerations apart from the bacteriological efficiency of the technique employed—time, and the state of the skin after the preparation. Some Continental chiropodists require their patients to soak their feet in an antiseptic foot-bath for ten minutes prior to treatment. For a chiropodist working single handed without a receptionist, this would entail a serious consumption of time during a day's work, apart from possibly having a rather unsatisfactory psychological effect on the patient. Also the skin would be left in a soggy state and most operators find that they prefer to work, in the majority of cases, on a dry foot rather than on one which has been recently soaked in hot water. The method of preparation must be quick and it must leave the skin pleasant to handle.

Two per cent of iodine in 70 per cent alcohol has been found to give satisfactory results when painted on to the skin and left for 15 seconds. "Hibitane" (I.C.I.), chlorhexidine digluconate or diacetate, has been the subject of extensive investigation along with other skin disinfectants. A 0·5 per cent chlorhexidine digluconate solution in 70 per cent alcohol has been found to have an action comparable with that of 2 per cent of iodine in 70 per cent alcohol. It attains its full effect very rapidly. One application by means of a swab is adequate though two swabbings are more effective than one. Traces of the antiseptic are left on the skin surface, and continue to exert a bactericidal effect. Sensitivity is rare.

The most commonly used method of preparing the skin of the foot for chiropody is to swab the foot either with a solvent or with a detergent. Alcohol, ethyl acetate, acetone and carbon tetrachloride are commonly used as solvents for this purpose. Each has its own particular advantages. Alcohol is cheap and pleasant to use, does not de-fat the skin too much and has a multiplicity of uses in chiropody. Alcohol does not dissolve rubber adhesive and, for this purpose, ethyl acetate, acetone, or carbon tetrachloride must be used as an auxiliary solvent. It has already been mentioned that these solvents vary in their efficiency with different types and ages of the plasters concerned. The solvents in general leave the skin in a pleasant condition to handle.

Of the detergents, solutions of sodium lauryl sulphate, laurolinium acetate, cetrimide, benzalkonium chloride or domiphen bromide are most commonly used, especially the last four which have germicidal as well as detergent properties. The detergents probably more readily remove the fat from the skin than do the solvents, and they may de-fat some skins too much. Cetrimide, benzalkonium chloride, domiphen bromide and laurolinium acetate, will act as germicides if they are in contact with the bacteria for a sufficient length of time, as is the case when they are allowed to dry on the skin. When working on the skin immediately following the application of a detergent, it can be difficult to obtain skin tension because the solution has left the skin in a slippery state. This is possibly due to the fact that they are employed in a somewhat curious way. Very few people would wash their hands in soap and water and then dry them without rinsing, and yet detergents, which act in the same general way as does soap, are used in precisely this manner. The foot is swabbed with the detergent and generally the detergent is allowed to remain on the skin without being rinsed away.

The pre-operative preparation of the skin of the operator's hands and the patient's feet consists of removing the transient bacterial population together with some of the resident population, generally by means of a solvent or a detergent. Quick-acting germicides may be used and some detergents also have a bactericidal action. For the hands, scrubbing with soap and water is the most satisfactory method.

CHAPTER VI

THE STERILIZATION OF INSTRUMENTS

IN the last chapter it was seen that the sterilization of the skin is difficult, if not impossible and that while a compromise is made by removing most of the pathogenic organisms, it cannot be claimed that the skin is left in a sterile condition. On the other hand it is quite easy to sterilize instruments by exposure to steam under pressure or by more sophisticated physical methods; expensive equipment is required but the actual procedure is simple enough. Instruments may also be sterilized by boiling at atmospheric pressure for twenty minutes, although this method will not kill bacterial spores. Unfortunately, exposure to steam or to boiling water of those instruments which are sharpened by stropping or honing hastens the corrosion of their cutting edges. The corrosion may be minimized by removing the dissolved oxygen, which is necessary for corrosion to take place, by the addition of sodium carbonate or sodium nitrite to the water.

The use of cold sterilization methods is not always appropriate where techniques involving soft tissue surgery are used. In these instances autoclaving of instruments is the indicated method of sterilization or instruments may be supplied in disposable pre-sterilized packs, or, where available, Central Sterilization Service may be used.

When considering the cold sterilization of instruments it must be remembered that the antiseptic in which the instruments are to be immersed will require time in which to act but, since each instrument is not in constant use, it should normally spend sufficient time in the antiseptic in the instrument dish to ensure adequate sterilization.

Cold sterilization of instruments takes place in three steps. These are:

1. The removal of gross contamination and the reduction of the number of micro-organisms present by the thorough mechanical cleansing of the instrument using a swab of cotton wool saturated with a solvent or detergent, generally the same preparation as that which is used in the preparation of the skin. In the case of files and burs and similar instruments, it may be necessary occasionally to use a wire brush, but they must be swabbed with a detergent whenever they are returned to the tray after use.

2. The instruments are *immersed* in a solution of a suitable anti-septic. It is important that the blades of instruments are completely immersed, both to ensure sterilization and also to minimize corrosion of the instrument.

3. The antiseptic is removed from the instrument, generally by wiping it with a swab of cotton wool soaked in alcohol or other solvent or detergent. If a detergent such as Teepol or Cetrimide is used before instruments are dried before putting them away for storage, the slight film of grease which is normally present may be removed and, lacking its protection, the instrument may rapidly become corroded.

The choice of antiseptic for the second stage is a matter for individual preference. Those most commonly used are:

1. *Chlorhexidine Solution* ("Hibitane", I.C.I., "Savlon Hospital Concentrate", I.C.I. [Savlon Hospital Concentrate contains in addition, Cetrimide 15 per cent]).

For the instrument tray a 0·1 per cent solution of "Hibitane" may be used. One gramme of sodium nitrite should be added to each litre of solution. Tablets of sodium nitrite are supplied with the "Hibitane" Concentrate. A separate tray containing a 0·5 per cent solution of "Hibitane" in alcohol and water may be used for the rapid sterilization of instruments or for instruments which have been grossly contaminated. The immersion time is given by the makers as 1–2 minutes. The solution is prepared by mixing 1 part of the Concentrate which contains 5 per cent of "Hibitane" with 1½ parts of distilled water and making up to 10 parts with Industrial Methylated Spirit.

The appropriate strengths of "Savlon Hospital Concentrate", are 1 in 200 in distilled water for instrument storage and 1 in 30 in Industrial Methylated Spirit for rapid sterilization.

2. *Chloroxylenol Solution* B.P.C. This is generally used in one of its proprietary forms, e.g.: "Dettol", "Ibcol", "Zant", etc. Some operators use the solution at full strength but a 2 per cent solution is to be preferred. "Instrument Dettol" is recommended for this purpose at 2 per cent strength. "Hycolin" (William Pearson) contains chlorocresols which are similar to chloroxylenols in their action. A 2 per cent dilution with added sodium nitrite is recommended for instrument sterilization.

"Novasapa" (Willows Francis) is a bactericidal solution containing a halogenated cresol, a tertiary amine and sodium citrate. It is used for the rapid cold-sterilization of instruments.

How far corrosion of sharp instruments can be avoided using the three-step cold sterilization method depends almost entirely on the care with which the technique is carried out. The first point to remember is that the blade of the instrument must be completely immersed in the antiseptic solution. The quickest way to bring about corrosion is to lay the instrument on top of a pad of saturated cotton wool, since this would produce the ideal conditions for corrosion, i.e. plenty of moisture and plenty of oxygen. If a piece of metal is partly immersed in water the spot most likely to suffer corrosion is the point where the metal enters the solution, where both oxygen and water are liberally available.

Another form of corrosion occurs when any metal is immersed in a solution which contains free ions. This is an electrolytic effect which results in the free ions reacting with small impurities in the metal of which the instrument is made. In effect small "batteries" are created and everyone is familiar with the corrosion which occurs at the terminals of a car battery.

A more recent problem has arisen from the appreciation of the risks of transmission of serum hepatitis type B. It is not possible to identify individual carriers of hepatitis type B antigen, although certain "at risk" classes may be identified. The virus may be transmitted by blood or other body fluids and therefore all instruments which have come into contact with any patient must be regarded as being contaminated. The routine cold sterilization process is not sufficient to eliminate the type B virus and therefore instruments have to be passed through an extra process which may be autoclaving, flash-boiling or treatment with a chemical such as glutaraldehyde.

The basic principle of the method suggested is that all instruments used on a particular patient should be isolated and subjected to the extra sterilization procedure before being returned to the instrument tray. This may involve keeping all instruments used on a patient in a separate dish or on a clean towel during a given treatment. The aim of the method is to prevent cross-infection or transmission of the virus. It is important that all instruments contaminated by serum, blood or pus should be washed thoroughly under running water before, for example, being immersed in glutaraldehyde if this be the "extra" method used.

CHAPTER VII

POST-OPERATIVE PROCEDURE —ANTISEPTIC TECHNIQUE

THE choice of post-operative procedure depends on whether the skin is apparently intact or whether there has been a breach in it sufficient to cause a haemorrhage. In either case, the object is the prevention of infection by a combination of three methods:

(1) A reduction in the number of pathogenic micro-organisms present.

(2) A reduction in the virulence of the pathogenic micro-organisms present.

(3) An increase in the resistance of the host.

The total disease-producing power of the micro-organisms depends upon their number and virulence, balanced against the resistance of the host and the state of this balance determines the establishment or the degree of severity of the infection.

Where the skin is apparently unbroken the chief danger of infection lies in the introduction of transient pathogenic micro-organisms via microscopic portals of entry caused by the removal of the stratum corneum. These pathogenic micro-organisms may be introduced via the operator's hands and instruments, via the dressings, or via the air. The prevention of the introduction of such organisms via the operator's hands and instruments has already been discussed in the previous two chapters. Air-borne infection cannot be ruled out but the risk can be lessened if the surgery is kept reasonably free from dust and is well ventilated. Infection via the dressings, which in the case of the intact skin are likely to be padding and strapping, is in many cases minimized by the inclusion of an antiseptic, generally zinc oxide, in the adhesive rubber plaster mass. It must be remembered that the adhesive is sticky and if it is exposed to the air for long periods it is likely to collect dust and germs even with the protective crinoline still in place. Care should be taken not to expose adhesive dressings and adhesive strappings to the air more than is absolutely necessary. If rolls of strapping are kept on a bar on the trolley as little strapping as possible should be left hanging from each spool.

Possibly the most important factor in post-operative procedure on the intact skin is the effect of adhesive plaster on the resistance of the skin to micro-organisms. The application of adhesive dressings must interfere with the secretory functions of the skin. The skin will be in a moist condition because the sweat cannot evaporate and the skin temperature raised by the retardation of evaporation and the prevention of loss of heat by radiation. There may be an accumulation of debris between the dressing and the skin. All these factors are in favour of the micro-organisms and tend to reduce the resistance of the skin to infection. Hence the importance of augmenting skin resistance by the application of a suitable antiseptic.

If no dressing is to be applied, then precautions are still very necessary since the skin will be exposed to contaminated hose and footwear.

The need for a post-operative antiseptic, then, is apparent, but what factors should influence the choice of antiseptic to be used? The antiseptic will be in contact with the skin for an indefinite period so that the concentration should be such that it does little damage to the skin cells. The most convenient method of applying the antiseptic is as a paint and it is desirable that the paint should dry quickly and be of such a colour that, while it does not obliterate the skin, the operator can see where the antiseptic has been applied. There will be no blood or other reactive organic material present so that an antiseptic which would be inactivated by the presence of blood may be employed. A greasy antiseptic is contra-indicated when adhesive dressings are to be used, although such an application could be made on a dry skin.

The most popular antiseptics in use today (not in order of popularity) are:

1. Chlorhexidine ("Hibitane", I.C.I.) as a 0·5 per cent solution in 70 per cent alcohol or as a 0·5 per cent aqueous solution. The disadvantage of these preparations is that, since they are virtually colourless when applied to the skin, it is not possible to identify easily the areas which have been covered.

2. Isopropyl alcohol 70 per cent. Again, this is colourless and is more effective as a wet dressing than as a paint.

3. Weak Iodine Solution B.P. This is one of the two most popular choices, the other being Compound Benzoin Tincture. Weak Iodine Solution acts quickly and is a suitable colour: some patients, however, show an idiosyncrasy to iodine.

4. Compound Benzoin Tincture B.P.C. is very popular because, when it has dried, it forms a film which acts as a flexible barrier

between skin and dressing and it does help to maintain the skin's resistance. Before it is completely dry it is tacky, which helps the adhesion of the pads on a greasy skin. Many operators find Compound Benzoin Tincture a completely satisfactory routine post-operative antiseptic.

5. A 1 per cent solution of cetrimide. This, applied as a paint and allowed to dry, is becoming increasingly popular. At first sight, it may be thought that this would lower the resistance of the skin by defatting it, but it must be remembered that it is applied as a paint and not as a detergent swab. It is difficult to ascertain whether there is an increase in the number of patients reacting unfavourably to plaster following the use of cetrimide, since the definition of what constitutes an unfavourable reaction varies very considerably from operator to operator.

Where there has been a haemorrhage the factors to be considered are rather different. The aim is still the same as that set out at the head of this chapter but with the addition that care must be taken not to lower the resistance of the host by destroying the leucocytes or interfering with the humoral chemistry.

It must be remembered that, here, it is a question of a wound which is not yet septic, but nevertheless, may have been invaded by pathogenic micro-organisms. When a clean wound is invaded by bacteria there is a two-hour lag phase before they start to proliferate and invade the tissues. Thus the antiseptic dressing has a two-hour start on the micro-organisms. It is not necessary to kill all the micro-organisms in a wound in order to prevent disease. Reduction in the number and virulence of the organisms will enable the resistance of the host to overcome them and it is important to realize that a bacteriostatic acts not only by inhibiting the growth of bacteria but, at the same time, also by reducing their virulence.

When an antiseptic is applied to a wound it will act on all the material with which it comes into contact. Some antiseptics, notably the antibiotics and the acridines, have an action which is directed against specific properties of the bacteria; that is to say, they have an effect on bacteria which they do not have on other tissue cells. They may have an effect on other tissue cells but it is different from that which they exert on the bacteria. The other antiseptics act in the same way on all the cells with which they come into contact. Thus, a protein precipitant will act on the tissue cells and blood cells as well as the bacterial ones. In fact, it has been clearly demonstrated that the leucocytes actually are more susceptible to the action of certain antiseptics than are the bacteria. This means that a certain concentration of an antiseptic will kill all the leucocytes in the blood but will not kill the bacteria present in the wound. Since leucocytes constitute an important defence of the body against infection, this means that the antiseptic has deprived it of its protection without, however, providing any substitute for the loss. The greatest advantage of the acridines as wound antiseptics is that, in bacteriostatic concentrations they do not interfere with leucocytic activity or with the process of repair. Many antiseptics lose their efficiency in the presence of organic matter and these are contraindicated as wound antiseptics.

Having chosen the antiseptic, the form in which it is used is another important consideration. If the tissues become waterlogged and macerated, their resistance is lowered. Maceration can be avoided in two ways: by applying a dressing that enables evaporation to take place freely or by using, where this is possible, an antiseptic in a spirit base.

The amino-acridines were probably the most generally used antiseptic on small clean wounds. Aminacrine as a 0·1 per cent solution in water or in 70 per cent isopropyl alcohol may be useful, depending on whether a drying action or a wet dressing is called for. The creams and emulsions of the acridines have now been largely superseded by such proprietary preparations as "Ponoxylan Gel", "Cicatrin" Powder and Cream, "Viacutan Emulsion" and Cetrimide Cream. Chlorhexidine ("Hibitane") is also widely used as a 0·1 per cent aqueous solution or as a cream in strengths from 0·1 to 1 per cent. If a dry dressing is required then "Cicatrin Powder" is useful and for prophylactic purposes hexachlorophane powders, such as "Sterzac Powder", have proved successful.

CHAPTER VIII

THE TREATMENT OF SEPTIC CONDITIONS

IN the last chapter wound-prophylaxis, that is the method by which wound infection may be prevented, was discussed. This chapter deals with wounds in which infection has been established. The objects of treatment are:

(1) To reduce the number of pathogenic organisms present:
   (a) by establishing drainage and removing them physically, and
   (b) by inhibiting their multiplication in the wound.
(2) To increase resistance to infection of the tissues.
(3) To encourage the healing of the wound and, at the same time, prevent further damage.

The treatment of septic conditions may be divided into five stages:
   (i) The establishment of drainage.
   (ii) The cleansing of the cavity.
   (iii) The application of heat.
   (iv) The application of an antiseptic dressing.
   (v) Resting the affected part.

To these procedures may be added the treatment of any predisposing factors. It may not be possible or desirable to carry out all five steps in every case. For instance, in many cases heat will not have to be applied, nor, when a lesion is draining by way of a sinus, is it always possible to clean out a cavity.

THE ESTABLISHMENT OF DRAINAGE

In many cases the establishment of drainage merely involves the removal of the superficial callus from a septic corn. After the removal of the thickened stratum corneum a shallow ulcer is left which can easily be cleaned out and dressed. In other cases, where there is a narrow track, or sinus, leading down to a larger cavity situated more deeply, this sinus must be cleared, using an enucleating technique, and it is often desirable to maintain drainage by means of a gauze wick. In some cases this wick may consist of a small piece of sterile gauze, in other cases it will be possible to introduce only a few strands of gauze into the sinus. This will help to maintain drainage and will also facilitate the clearing of the sinus on the return visit.

In some cases the condition is not sufficiently developed for drainage to be established and the sepsis is sometimes said to be "unripe", an unscientific but nevertheless apt description. In this event, a prolonged application of moist heat is indicated. This has the effect of speeding up the inflammatory process, encouraging the formation of the enzyme trypsin, which digests the skin, and of macerating and weakening the epidermis so that the enclosed pocket of pus is enabled to break through the skin at the weakest point. The heat is applied by means of a kaolin poultice, hot compresses or hot foot-bath. Hot compresses and foot-baths need frequent repetition and in the case of the former the patient must be able to replace his own dressing or have someone who is able to do this for him. If a patient is not able to have frequent foot-baths or compresses a kaolin poultice should be used. As an alternative to the application of moist heat Basilicon Ointment (Colophony Ointment B.P.C.) may be applied. It should be spread thickly on lint and then applied to the affected area. Once drainage has been established either a saline dressing or a dressing of Morison's Paste (Magnesium Sulphate Paste B.P.C.) may be used. The Magnesium Sulphate Paste, by its osmotic action, "draws" the condition by removing water from the tissues. These techniques are employed when the inflammatory process has not reached its fullest intensity.

CLEANSING THE CAVITY

The cleansing of the cavity depends on its size, shape and accessibility. The cavity may be cleaned by swabbing with a solution of 1 per cent cetrimide in water, 0·33 per cent Hibitane in water, normal saline, or chlorine antiseptics such as Eusol or Dakin's solution. If a spray is used it should be used with great caution. The use, of Hydrogen Peroxide Solution as a cleansing agent has recently been questioned, since it may be toxic when it is absorbed. Nevertheless, it may be useful in cases of acute sepsis. Its use on chronic ulceration is best avoided. The bubbling action of the Hydrogen Peroxide coming into contact with infected material will break up the pus to a certain degree and will facilitate its removal by a gentle sponging with a sterile swab saturated with Hydrogen Peroxide Solution. An alternative method of removing pus, etc., from the wound is to use a foot-bath. The method will be described in the next section since this is also a method of applying heat.

THE APPLICATION OF HEAT

When dealing with a septic case, heat may conveniently be applied:

(1) As a foot-bath which gives a large quantity of heat for a short period.

(2) As infra-red irradiations, which have the advantage of not pressing on the wound, and with which the risk of infecting other parts of the foot are less than is the case with a foot-bath.

(3) By means of poultices which exert a mild but lasting action.

There are certain contraindications to the application of heat. Patients who are known diabetics and have peripheral neuropathy should not be allowed to use foot-baths at home. Patients with severe arterio-sclerosis should not as a general rule be given heat to the extremities. This does not exclude a warm foot-bath at say 38° C. (100° F.) being used to help cleanse a wound.

A hot foot-bath may be either antiseptic or effervescent. Since the virtue of a foot-bath lies in the quantity of heat which it makes available it is essential to use plenty of water. (It must be understood that these remarks refer specifically to the use of foot-baths in the treatment of septic conditions.)

It will be found that a foot-bath which will hold about two gallons of water is a convenient size to handle and it should be half filled, i.e. with 1 gallon (or 5 litres) of water. For an antiseptic foot-bath given in the surgery, 2 ounces (or 60 grammes) of Chloroxylenol Solution, or 2 ounces of common salt (Sodium Chloride), should be added to the 1 gallon of water which should be given at a temperature of 46° C. (115° F.). If a foot-bath is being given at home the patient should be instructed to fill a large bowl with comfortably warm water and to add to it a handful of household salt.

For an effervescent foot-bath two substances are added to the water of the bath which will interact to release a supply of carbon dioxide. This will tend to break up the pus and will also create a marked hyperaemia. There are several methods of preparing such baths. Sodium bicarbonate may be dissolved in the water and crystals of tartaric acid added to it so that the stream of bubbles of carbon dioxide then liberated may be directed on to the septic cavity. For the official Effervescent Bath sodium bicarbonate and sodium bisulphate are the ingredients (see also Carbon Dioxide, page 159). The foot-bath should be given for as long a period as is convenient, up to about twenty minutes, and the temperature of the water should be maintained by the addition of hot water.

Infra-red irradiations may be used instead of a foot-bath, and may be followed by the application of Kaolin Poultice which, of course, may also be used immediately after the cavity has been cleaned. A kaolin poultice may be used not only to establish drainage when the sepsis has not yet come to a head but also in cases when the septic condition is well established. Care must be taken to prevent the poultice from "plugging" the opening of a septic cavity as this might interfere with its drainage. Besides being a method for the application of heat, Kaolin Poultice will also absorb pus and serum from an open lesion.

AFTER-DRESSING: THE ENCOURAGEMENT OF THE HEALING PROCESS

The choice of antiseptic for dressing a septic wound will depend on the state of the ulcer which is left after the pus has been cleared. In any case the antiseptic must be one which is efficient in the presence of pus and other organic material (see also page 22 ff.) but is not so caustic as to cause further damage to the tissue cells. As it is not convenient to identify the infecting organism in every case of sepsis an antiseptic which has a wide antibacterial spectrum should be chosen, for example Polynoxylin 10 per cent ("Ponoxylan", Berk Pharm.) or Methargen ("Viacutan", Ward, Blenkinsop). For a very dirty septic wound chlorine antiseptics are still widely used. Either inorganic or organic preparations may be employed. The chlorine has the effect of stimulating the flow of lymph and of rendering necrosed tissue more easily soluble in tissue fluids by forming soluble chloramines. Eusol and Dakin's Solution are popular inorganic chlorine preparations and chloramine and dichloramine may be used where an organic preparation is required. The organic chlorine preparations are less irritant than the inorganic ones.

A soggy ulcer may be treated with 70 per cent alcohol as an after dressing or with a solution of one of the acridines, e.g. proflavine or aminacrine, in spirit. The soggy type of indolent ulcer may be treated with "Aserbine" (Malic acid) or with "Ponoxylan" Gel which is not only a very powerful antiseptic but is also a corticomimetic. A 1 per cent solution of Brilliant Green may be used but Crystal Violet is contra-indicated in septic conditions generally. These dyes are not widely used because of their obliterating colour.

Where an ulcer is dry following the removal of pus, "Cicatrin" powder may be used followed by a Tulle Gras dressing, or Cream of Proflavine or Cream of Aminacrine may be employed. Again "Ponoxylan Gel" or "Viacutan" are very useful in this type of wound. When the pus is very stiff the Creams of the Acridines may be used, with Ichthammol Glycerin, Magnesium Sulphate Paste or "Viacutan Emulsion" as alternatives. If, on the other hand, the pus is thin and watery a 1 per cent solution of Brilliant Green or "Viacutan Emulsion" may be chosen and the wound kept as dry as possible. It is a mistake to persist too long with any one kind of treatment. Bacteria may quickly become insensitive or even resistant to a particular drug and a change may produce good results. Changes should be made every few days unless the condition is showing signs of good progress.

REST

When the wound has been dressed, the affected part must be rested as much as possible. This is of paramount importance. Complete physical rest is the ideal but where this is not possible the removal of all pressure from the part must be maintained by padding, cutting the shoes or by other methods, such as wearing a carpet slipper on the affected foot.

Ulcers which are not caused by sepsis are sometimes encountered on the foot. The ulcer produced by the action of caustics used in the treatment of warts is one example; this is dealt with under the treatment of warts. Pressure ulcers and ulcers due to circulatory disorders are also seen, particularly in patients suffering from diabetes and other diseases showing arterio-sclerotic changes. The prime objects in treating such ulcers is to prevent infection, remove any trauma and use preparations that are stimulating and will encourage the formation of granulation tissue.

In the early stages a septic case should be seen every day, if this is at all possible, or at least every other day. As the acute condition subsides the return periods should be gradually lengthened. In the majority of infected cases, the infection occurs because a portal of entry has been provided for pathogenic organisms, and any prophylactic measures taken must be steps to prevent a similar situation arising. An example is the case of a relaxed nail sulcus which has predisposed to a septic ingrown toe-nail; prophylactic measures should in this case be directed towards hardening the nail sulcus. In other cases of infection, there may be a septic focus remote from the foot and a septic condition on the foot may then occur on a *locus resisentiae minoris*. If infection takes place for no apparent reason, or if infection occurs repeatedly, the patient should be encouraged to seek medical advice.

CHAPTER IX

THE ARREST OF HAEMORRHAGE

NORMALLY, when blood is shed from the vessels it coagulates by the following mechanism. When the blood platelets come into contact with a water-wettable[1] surface they coagulate, disintegrate and liberate an enzyme, thrombokinase. This substance is produced also by damaged blood and tissue cells. In the presence of calcium ions, thrombokinase converts prothrombin (a substance present in the blood plasma) into thrombin. Thrombin converts fibrinogen, which is also present in blood plasma, into an insoluble protein, fibrin, which forms the blood clot.

The minor haemorrhages encountered in chiropody may be stopped either by means of a styptic drug or by the use of some mechanical styptic such as cotton wool, gelatin sponge or oxidized cellulose. The action of these is to break up the blood into tiny drops and to provide a large water-wettable surface, thus accelerating the normal clotting process while, at the same time, limiting to some extent the rate of flow. The haemostatic drugs may have a direct constricting action on the blood vessels, or they may act by precipitating the cell protein, thus forming a barrier that prevents the flow of blood, which then clots normally underneath the barrier. Unfortunately, this method devitalizes other cells in the region of the wound and may delay healing, as well as providing ideal conditions for promoting infection. The most commonly used methods for the arrest of haemorrhage in chiropody are the following:

1. The application of Ferric Chloride Solution or a 10 per cent Solution of Silver Nitrate. Both of these medicaments act by precipitating protein and forming a barrier to the flow of blood from an abrasion, and it is therefore important that the barrier should be formed as near to the source of the haemorrhage as possible. It is useless to apply one of these medicaments to a small drop of blood.

---

[1] Water-wettable means exactly what it suggests: able to be wet by water. A very large number of surfaces are not water-wettable. If, for example, the hand is dipped into water and then withdrawn it will be noticed that the water has not wet the skin, but lies in droplets on the surface. If the skin is first smeared with petroleum jelly the effect is even more marked. Paper of most types is water-wettable, otherwise it could not be written on with ink, or painted on with water colour paints.

The only effect would be that the outside layer of the droplet would be precipitated and form a skin which would be very rapidly broken.

Before applying the drug all blood must be wiped away from the abrasion so that the ferric chloride, or silver nitrate, solution can reach the tissues surrounding the abrasion, precipitate the protein and form a block. If there is a flap of tissue the styptic must be introduced underneath the flap in order to reach the tissues surrounding the wound.

Only very small quantities of ferric chloride are required and it is not necessary to drop the solution itself on to the haemorrhage. It should be remembered that ferric chloride is also caustic. The following method is suggested. Place one drop of Ferric Chloride Solution on a swab of cotton wool. Take a second cotton wool swab and bring it into contact with the ferric chloride on the first swab. It is often convenient for the second swab to be wrapped round the end of a tapered wooden applicator before it is brought into contact with the Ferric Chloride Solution. This facilitates accurate application which is essential to this method. The second swab of wool will be almost dry but will be stained yellow by the ferric chloride. The flowing blood or any accumulation of blood is wiped away from the bleeding-point and the second, almost dry, swab is pressed firmly over the bleeding-point. This method is far more effective than dropping Ferric Chloride Solution on to the bleeding-point and also is far less messy and painful.

The application of a styptic is generally painful but the pain can be reduced if an analgesic is applied first or is incorporated with the styptic. A styptic of the latter type is:

R. Tannic acid powder   20
    Benzocaine   10
    Starch   to   100

Solutions of alum, copper sulphate or ferric sulphate may be used instead of solutions of ferric chloride or silver nitrate. It should be noted that the rate of sepsis following the application of silver nitrate as a haemostatic appears to be higher than is the case with most other styptics. Ferric chloride is to be preferred if a protein precipitant is to be used.

Many small bleeding points can be controlled by applying a swab of sterile cotton wool with firm digital pressure. The swab may be saturated with "Hibitane" or other readily available antiseptic.

With a rather more severe haemorrhage, for instance if a wart has inadvertently been sliced, the following method may be used. Take a foot-bath and fill with 1 gallon (or 5 litres) of water at 46° C.

(115° F.) and add 2 fl. oz. (60 ml.) Solution of Chloroxylenol. Immerse the patient's foot in the bath and maintain the temperature of the water until bleeding ceases. The temperature of the water will speed up the clotting of the blood and the water itself, by nullifying the effect of gravity, will prevent the blood from flowing away from the wound and will so enable a clot to form over the abraded blood vessels. An antiseptic after-dressing will, of course, be required.

A 1:1,000 Solution of Adrenaline has a direct action on the blood vessels by causing vasoconstriction. A haemorrhage which has been arrested with adrenaline may be dressed with any of the usual wound prophylactics.

There are also available for effecting haemostasis commercial products containing calcium alginate, e.g. "Calgitex". These are available as either wool, gauze and ribbon gauze. They work on the principle that when blood or serum come into contact with the alginate wool or gauze, it swells and assumes a gel-like form. The gel forms an enormous number of points at which clotting can occur. In addition, calcium ions, which as mentioned are essential for the formation of the enzyme thrombin, are released and thereby increase the clotting process. The wool form has the advantage that it can be used with digital pressure if desired.

CHAPTER X

THE TREATMENT OF ASEPTIC INFLAMMATION

IN an earlier chapter it was pointed out that inflammation is a process and not a state and is generally continuous, with, and inseparable from, the process of repair. Inflammation has been defined as the succession of changes which occur in the living tissue when it is injured. This is a clear enough definition, and it was John Hunter who reintroduced the important concept, that inflammation could be initiated by any insult, for instance, pressure, friction, heat, cold, etc. It is the treatment of this type of inflammation that is here being considered. Aseptic inflammation will produce the "triple response", but the treatment differs fundamentally from the treatment of bacterial inflammation in that:

(1) The process of phagocytosis plays a comparatively minor role, since there are no bacteria to attack and ingest; the phagocytes have to deal only with damaged cells.

(2) The role of the exudate is less important in that antibodies and antitoxins are not required.

Inflammation due to trauma is common in the foot and the fundamental treatment is rest in the widest sense of the term, including not only the physical rest of the inflamed tissue, but also the removal of the source of irritation. The inflammatory reaction does play a defensive role in that the part concerned will be painful and the patient will naturally try not to use it. Many cases of traumatic inflammation in the foot are due to repeated minor traumata caused by some mechanical defect in the functioning of the foot, and the resting of the part in such a way that the patient is able to continue his normal activities is the greatest skill of the chiropody practitioner.

From the study of the introductory chapter on inflammation, it will be clear that there are two phases in the early stages of the process, the first phase being one of active hyperaemia, with much exudation, and the second, one of stasis in both blood vessels and tissues. The treatment which should accompany rest in these two phases is obviously quite different. Because the first phase is limited in its usefulness when bacteria are not present, it is desirable to restrict it as far as possible; the use of cold and/or astringent lotions is, therefore, indicated. In the second phase, it is important that resolution rather than organization should take place so that the absorption of the static exudate should be encouraged by the use of heat and rubefacients. Finally, steps may have to be taken to restore the normal function of the tissues, for example movement and exercises in the case of synovitis of a joint. When ulceration has occurred the repair process must be assisted and encouraged.

While the principles of treatment of aseptic inflammation may appear, in themselves, to be quite simple, the manifestations of aseptic inflammation are diverse and complicated. For instance, there is a vast apparent difference between the inflammation produced by a single major trauma such as the violent stubbing of a great toe or the sudden wrenching of an ankle joint, and the inflammation produced by repeated minor traumata or by continuous overstrain of some of the ligaments of the foot.

Probably the most common type of inflammation found in the feet arises from repeated minor traumata, unavoidable in the natural process of locomotion, where the tissues concerned are unable to withstand the stress and strain to which they are subjected. All degrees of inflammation are encountered in the feet, as will be seen when the inflammation of specific structures is discussed. The broad principles of treatment are the same in every case; rest, combined with the use of cooling and astringent medicaments in the phase of effusion and of rubefacients in the phase of stasis.

SPRAINS, STRAINS AND MUSCLE FATIGUE

A sprain is the wrenching of a joint with injury to its surrounding structures without the luxation (dislocation) of bones, i.e. a sprain is an inflammation which is caused by a single major trauma. The exudative phase of inflammation is very marked and there is generally a good deal of pain. In the early stages of a sprain, the treatment is the application of cold or cooling lotions, together with firm bandaging to control the swelling and to immobilize the joint. Lead Lotion, Evaporating and Lead Lotion, used undiluted, are commonly used by saturating several layers of lint in the chosen lotion and bandaging them firmly into position under a layer of cotton wool. The layer of cotton wool eliminates the danger of the bandage cutting into the flesh if further swelling should take place. The application of ice packs is useful if these are available. If the condition does not respond rapidly to treatment, medical advice should be sought. As soon as the exudative phase is complete and the severe pain has subsided, active and passive movements should be encouraged, together with the application of heat or a rubefacient liniment such as Methyl Salicylate Liniment or, more commonly, White Liniment or Turpentine Liniment. Bandaging and strapping of the joint may be necessary for some time but should be dispensed with gradually. In patients with a tendency repeatedly to "turn" or "rick" a joint, the matter should be treated as a mechanical problem.

A strain, in the sense in which it is being discussed here, may be defined as the result of the inability of the tissues concerned to stand up to the stresses to which they are subjected. Although the term acute foot strain is used in the sense of severe foot strain, a strain is essentially chronic in nature—the stresses are either continuous or repeated. The treatment in the first instance is rest and the long-term treatment must aim at discovering and correcting any underlying dysfunction of the foot, by modifying the transmission of body weight on the component parts of the foot, where there is some anatomical abnormality; by re-education of muscle, where there is muscle imbalance; by correction of posture and gait, and attention to footwear, etc. Since the strain is long-standing, the local treatment will be the relief of congestion. This may be accomplished by the use of heat but a better result is often obtained by the use of alternate hot and cold foot-baths, especially in the causes of muscle fatigue. The use of rubefacients is rare in foot strain. Sometimes the swabbing of the skin with spirit or Spiritus Pedibus is recommended followed by the application of an astringent dusting-powder. The success of this treatment is probably due to its effect as a local treatment for the slight hyperidrosis which frequently accompanies a strained foot. In severe cases of foot strain, rest in bed, if only for a long weekend, is highly desirable. This may be followed by rest by means of padding and strapping, together with the application of heat from a luminous source. Hot wax baths are also useful in severe cases. Exercises are contra-indicated in cases of strained feet until the symptoms have completely subsided.

SYNOVITIS AND TENOSYNOVITIS

Synovitis and tenosynovitis may occur as the result of a single major trauma or of repeated minor traumata, and the same general principles may be applied as for other types of aseptic inflammation. In the acute stage cooling lotions may be applied together with rest and, following the subsidence of swelling and pain, rubefacients may be applied. The best rubefacient in these cases is undoubtedly heat from an infra-red or a radiant heat lamp; this may be followed by an application of Iodine Ointment, Non-staining, or iodine oil with or without methyl salicylate. In some cases liniments such as Turpentine Liniment or Methyl Salicylate Liniment may be used. The restoration of a full range of movement at the joint concerned is an important feature of the later stages of treatment. The identification and removal of the cause of the synovitis or tenosynovitis is extremely important. This is generally a problem of foot mechanics.

BURSITIS

Perhaps the most common manifestation of aseptic inflammation which the chiropodist is called upon to treat is a traumatic bursitis. Both anatomical and adventitious bursae may be affected. In severe cases, the bursal sac is distended with fluid and the part is very hot, red and painful. The fluid may sometimes track to the skin in order to find an outlet at the surface. In this stage such cooling and astringent lotions as Aluminium Acetate Solution diluted to half strength or, occasionally, Lead Lotion may be used. As an alternative, an application of warm Kaolin Poultice will often give a very good result and, in cases where a track has been formed, an application of warm Magnesium Sulphate Paste may be very effective. Active steps must be taken to relieve pressure and friction on the bursa. Once a track has been formed care must be taken to prevent secondary infection from taking place. Generally, with the relief of pressure the condition subsides quite rapidly to a stage where rubefacients, including heat, may be used. Iodine Ointment, Non-staining, is a useful rubefacient since, if necessary, it may be used as a "buffer"-ointment in a cavity pad. Methyl salicylate may be incorporated in the Iodine Ointment and this acts as an analgesic as well as being a very powerful rubefacient. As an alternative, the skin over the bursa may be painted with Iodine Solution, Strong, either alone or with Compound Benzoin Tincture.

It has been mentioned that the fluid in the bursa may force its way out by a track to the surface of the skin. In course of time, the walls of the track may become organized or fibrotic, particularly at the opening of the track at the surface. Before the track will close and heal, this fibrotic tissue must be destroyed by means of suitable medicaments. Silver nitrate, 40 per cent solution, is popular because of its localized and rather superficial action. The solution is painted round the orifice of the track and left for up to fourteen days, after which the coagulum is carefully dissected away. This treatment should be repeated at fairly frequent intervals until the track has been obliterated. An alternative method is to apply a drop or two of pure phenol for two minutes and then to wash out the track with spirit. Rectified spirit has also been used for its dehydrating action in place of silver nitrate or phenol.

Although it is nearly always desirable to close the track leading from a bursa in order to minimize the risk of infection from the outside, it is quite another matter whether an attempt should be made to destroy a bursal sac itself. Sometimes the contents of a bursal sac which has been inflamed becomes fibrotic and the bursa becomes permanently distended and unsightly. The patient, in these cases, usually complains of the unsightliness of the bursa rather than of pain. All bursae in the first instance perform a definite and useful protective function and before it is decided to destroy a bursal sac, it is absolutely essential to ensure that the part which the bursa was protecting is no longer in need of such protection and is not likely to require such special protection in future. If the operator still decides that it is desirable to destroy the bursal sac, the same methods may be used as for the track leading down to the bursa. It must be emphasized that a bursa is *locus resistentiae minoris* and is particularly liable to become infected, and that the application of irritants to the sac will increase rather than diminish the risk of infection. In cases of chronic, post-inflammatory enlargement of a bursa the energetic use of rubefacients will often promote some absorption of fluid with diminution in the size of the bursa. Iodine Solution, Strong, is particularly effective and may be combined with the use of pressure strappings.

CHILBLAINS

Chilblains may be considered under the general heading of aseptic inflammation and, once again, it is necessary to have a clear picture of the physiological and pathological processes involved in order to establish the principles of treatment. The blood supply to the skin, in addition to supplying it with nourishment and providing protection in the inflammatory response, also plays an important part in regulating the amount of heat lost by the body by radiation. In cold weather, in order to minimize the amount of heat lost by the body to its surroundings, the arterioles in the skin become constricted and the skin becomes cold. Since the skin is cold, the metabolic rate of the surface tissues is diminished and generally there is no abnormal de-oxygenation of the blood. Normally, when the body's surroundings become warmer, for instance when an individual comes from a cold environment into a warm room, the arterioles relax and more blood flows through the superficial arterial plexus. In some cases the relaxation of the arterioles in a certain area is delayed, with the result that when the superficial tissues become warmer and their metabolic rate increases there is not a sufficient supply of nourishment, the blood becomes excessively de-oxygenated and the part becomes cyanosed. If, at this stage, the arterioles relax no permanent damage will have resulted to the tissues, but if the circulation continues to be restricted the metabolites, the waste products of tissue metabolism, will not be carried away but will accumulate in the area. This causes the capillaries to become more permeable and there will be a local increase in the amount of tissue fluid but, since this tissue fluid is derived from static blood, it will soon be used up by the tissues and there will be a further accumulation of metabolites. If the chilling continues local damage is done to the tissues by the accumulated metabolites and a potential inflammation is set up. The inflammation is "potential" because the tissues cannot respond with the normal inflammatory process while the arterioles remain constricted. This state of affairs constitutes the chilblain lesion. When the inflammation is established, the arterioles become dilated and the familiar cycle of events occurs with redness, heat, swelling and pain in the form of an intense itching. Since there is an abnormality of the blood vessels in the area and since there is the likelihood of fresh exposure to the exciting cause—cold—the exudative stage of the inflammation is frequently prolonged.

Thus, in chilblains there is:

1. A stage at which, owing to abnormality in the small blood vessels or in their nerve supply, the supply of blood to the tissues is insufficient to meet their metabolic requirements: metabolites accumulate in the tissues, and tissue cells are damaged. This is sometimes called the cyanotic stage because of the bluish appearance given to the skin by the de-oxygenated blood.

2. At a later stage the damaged tissues evoke the inflammatory response which goes through (a) the hyperaemic phase, and (b) the congestive stage of inflammation.

It is obvious that in the early or cyanotic stages of chilblains the object of treatment will be the relaxation of the arterioles and for this purpose mild rubefacients are generally used, particularly those which exert a mild lasting effect. Iodine is again a popular choice, either as Iodine Ointment, Non-staining, or as Iodine Solution, Weak, half and half with Compound Benzoin Tincture. Certain of the rubefacients also exert a mild analgesic action that relieves the itching which may be associated with this stage of chilblains. Methyl salicylate, clove oil, camphor, capsicum, histamine, menthol and acetylcholine have all been used as ingredients for chilblain remedies. Ichthammol, 10 per cent in flexible collodion, or as a 10 per cent ointment, and coal tar, as Coal Tar Paste, are also used in the early stages of chilblains, although these are possibly more appropriate to the broken stage. If heat is used as a rubefacient in the early stages of chilblains, it should be employed with caution and the application should be quite mild. Frequently several medicaments having rubefacient or analgesic properties are combined to make a chilblain remedy and there is a number of sound proprietary preparations on the market.

The rubefacient and analgesic paints and ointments may also be used in the inflammatory stage of chilblains but in this stage a better result is often obtained by the use of cooling and astringent lotions such as Calamine Lotion, Burow's Solution, Witch Hazel Solution or Lead Lotion. As with the other types of inflammation discussed, there is an exudative phase and a phase of stasis. In the exudative phase, the cooling lotions are indicated and the rubefacients in the phase of stasis. Contrast foot-baths are useful when the crisis of the inflammatory stage has passed.

Because chilblains occur on sites where the circulation is poor, and very often on sites which are subjected to external traumata, it quite frequently happens that the inflammatory reaction does not give sufficient protection and that local necrosis of tissue takes place. The chilblains are then described as "broken chilblains". The treatment of broken chilblains is to apply antiseptics which are mildly stimulating, antipruritic and anti-inflammatory. Preparations of "Ponoxylan Gel", Ichthammol and Coal Tar are often employed with good effect, as are also preparations of Peru Balsam. Dressings which tend to lead to sogginess of the tissues are to be avoided. Magnesium Sulphate Paste and warm Kaolin Poultice may be used to relieve the congestion and swelling of broken chilblains.

It is known that the exciting cause of chilblains is cold, particularly damp cold, but the predisposing causes of the condition are obscure. A number of factors, such as calcium deficiency and endocrine imbalance, have been suggested as playing a part. Prophylactic measures may be taken to deal with the supposed predisposing causes of the condition, and to stimulate the blood flow towards the superficial tissues by means of the internal administration of nicotinic acid and its derivatives. These measures are the concern of the medical practitioner. Prophylactic measures may also be directed against the exciting cause by such steps as the wearing of warm hosiery and the avoidance of exposure to cold. The chiropodist should advise patients on these points.

An important consideration in the treatment of chilblains is their after effects on the skin. Where necrosis of the tissues has occurred some degree of scarring is to be expected. Chilblains frequently occur on sites exposed to friction and pressure and the scarring gives rise to very painful lesions, which are often labelled "vascular corns" and which are very difficult to treat successfully. The use of an emollient cream by the patient for a considerable period following an attack of chilblains will help to keep the skin supple and prevent it from hardening. Measures to increase the superficial circulation, such as vigorous scrubbing with soap and water and drying with a rough towel, will assist in improving the texture of the skin and should be carried out during the summer and autumn months.

ULCERATION FOLLOWING ASEPTIC INFLAMMATION

Where the outcome of aseptic inflammation is ulceration, the ulcer, once it has been exposed to the air, will not be free from bacteria. In general, the treatment of such ulcers is by the use of antiseptics which have a mildly stimulating effect. In some cases, it may be sufficient to paint the ulcer with a layer of Compound Benzoin Tincture, Flexible Collodion or other plastic dressing and healing will take place underneath the protective layer of the medicament. It is important to avoid sogginess and, therefore, one must consider the base of any medicaments applied, that is, are they miscible with the exudate. Oil-in-water creams, gels such as "Ponoxylan" and "Viacutan Emulsion" can be used with good effect, but the water-in-oil creams and ointments are contra-indicated. If the acridines are being used a solution of an acridine in spirit is preferable to a cream. "T.C.P." at full strength is a useful preparation, or it may be diluted with spirit to half strength. If an ulcer shows signs of becoming chronic, the underlying reason must be discovered and, if possible, rectified. Local treatment may be by the use of preparations of coal tar, ichthammol or Povidone-iodine. Zinc Sulphate Lotion is a satisfactory astringent lotion. If the ulcer is of very long standing, a smear of Scarlet Red Ointment round its edges will stimulate granulation. A special case of an ulcer following aseptic inflammation is the breakdown of tissue after the use of acids in the treatment of warts. This is discussed under the heading of the treatment of warts (see page 104).

CHAPTER XI

THE TREATMENT OF CORNS AND CALLUS

THE rational treatment of corns and callus is still seriously hampered by a lack of detailed knowledge of mechanisms by which the skin produces these excrescences. Certain facts are established:

1. Corn and callus may occur where skin suffers a kneading action between bone and some other solid resistance which may be the shoe, another bone, or the ground. Callus and corn may occur also where the skin is trapped between the upper and insole of the shoe.

2. Such kneading may or may not produce corn and callus. It seems that certain skins show a predisposition to produce callosities and other skins do not have such a tendency. No explanation has yet been advanced as to why this should be so.

3. Thickening of the stratum corneum may be produced by factors other than mechanical stresses. Thickening of the stratum corneum means that skin cells are produced at a rate faster than they are shed. Such a thickening might result either from an increase in the number of cells produced in the stratum germinativum or from a slowing down of the rate at which cells are shed by desquamation from the stratum corneum. The weight of the evidence accumulated in recent years now suggests that the former hypothesis may be rejected.

Both the process of keratinization and also the resulting product has been shown to vary quite widely in different regions of the skin. It has also been shown that different physical conditions such as pressure may modify both process and product. Keratinization is now regarded not merely as being the death of cells, but as an active process whereby the skin cells are converted into the strong inert protective covering of the body. Keratinization is a purposeful physiological activity controlled by enzymes catalysing the processes which convert the cytoplasmic contents of the skin cells into keratin. In the "normal" process of keratinization, the cell nucleus is lost as well as the major part of the cell content. Only the outer part of the cell finally becomes completely keratinized. The rest of the cell is broken down by enzymes present in the granular region into water-

97

soluble substances which disappear. The result is a pliable network of keratin. In contrast to this form of keratinization, on the palms and the soles, the nuclei of the epidermal cells are lost but most of the cell contents become keratinized. Because most of the cell is keratinized, the keratin formed consists of what might be described as small "bricks" of keratin, in contrast to the basket weave of the keratin produced in other areas. The keratin thus produced is much less pliable but is a tougher and thicker structure, better able to stand up to the greater wear and tear imposed on the hands and the feet. Other modifications of the keratinization process occur in the production of the hair and nails.

A great deal has been learned of the detailed biochemistry of the various keratinization processes, although it cannot be claimed that these are by any means fully understood. Few suggestions have been made as to means whereby abnormalities of the resulting product might be prevented or corrected. Therefore, at the present time, there is not room in a book dealing with therapeutics for a review of these processes. This is not to underestimate their importance. The essential point is that keratinization is an active, positive physiological process, which may be modified by environmental factors such as pressure and stress.

The mechanical cause of a particular corn or callus can generally be identified and, in many cases, corrected or at least palliated, and the removal of the mechanical cause should always be one of the first considerations in treating these conditions. There are, however, many cases where either the mechanical cause cannot be identified or, more commonly, where it cannot be rectified, and in these cases the treatment of the local lesions is of paramount importance. While the treatment of corn and callus is still based on empirical ideas it must be emphasized that the treatment of these conditions should be active and positive. Quite rightly, the term "cut and come again" is anathema to every self-respecting chiropodist. Many cases of corn and callus can be cured, given knowledge and skill on the part of the chiropodist and a reasonable degree of co-operation on the part of the patient. The aim of treatment is to restore the skin to its normal texture, and this is achieved by analysis of the causative factors and their elimination or their modifications. The question of the mechanical causes of corn and callus again lies outside the scope of this work.

The local treatment falls into two parts: first, the removal of the thickened stratum corneum, and secondly, the restoration of the skin to its normal texture and resilience. Complete removal of the cornified tissue is essential, and it is also important to prevent the accumulation of a thickened stratum corneum in order to prevent pressure keratinization occurring in the deeper layers. If the tissues are to return to normal, complete removal of the cornified tissues is essential and very frequent treatment, possibly every 2 or 3 days initially, may be necessary in order to prevent a build-up of cornified tissue.

For the removal of the thickened stratum corneum and of the nucleus of corns, nothing can take the place of a sound operating technique using sharp instruments. It has already been stressed that the removal of every scrap of thickened stratum corneum is fundamental to the treatment of corn and callus. To have to resort to the use of salicylic acid, except in a few unusual cases, is an admission of failure of technique, although salicylic acid may profitably be used to soften deep corns which are difficult to remove painlessly.

Certain types of callus, notably rather vascular types, do respond well to the application of a 20–40 per cent pyrogallic acid plaster. A return period of from fourteen to twenty-one days is suggested for this method. The use of vitamin E cream, wheat germ oil, either alone or in conjunction with pyrogallic acid ointment, has been employed successfully in the treatment of fibrous corns, and in particular of very deep plantar corns embedded in a mass of fibrous tissue. It seems probable that vitamin E cream has an effect on the disorder of collagen in the dermis which is so often associated with deep corns. Indeed it has been suggested that in this type of corn the primary disorder lies in the dermis and that the corn is secondary to it. It is suggested that a chronic inflammation may be set up in the dermis resulting in the formation of fibrous tissue, which binds down a certain area of skin tightly to the fascia, and this area becomes a site of a deep fibrous corn.

The removal of extremely hard callus on the plantar metatarsal area or around the heel—the type of thickening which is often referred to as *hyperkeratosis*, as distinct from *callus* (the writer sees no justification for the restriction of the term hyperkeratosis to such conditions), may be faciliated by the application of crude soft soap. The technique is to immerse the foot in a foot-bath until it is well soaked and then to rub soft soap into the affected parts. The foot is then again immersed in the foot-bath and is taken out after 5 minutes' immersion, the surface moisture is absorbed with towels, using a squeezing and not a rubbing action, then more soft soap is applied and the whole covered with lint and elastoplast. The patient should return in 7 days still wearing the dressings. Crude soft soap contains a certain amount of free potassium hydroxide which softens the hardened stratum corneum. It also contains fats which serve as an emollient. It will be realized that this may be a somewhat inconvenient form of treatment from the patient's point of view, nevertheless it does achieve good results and the severity of these cases may justify this drastic form of treatment.

After the removal of the thickened stratum corneum, there are, in general, four courses open for the local treatment of the lesion:

(1) An antiseptic paint.

(2) An astringent or a caustic.

(3) An emollient.

(4) Stimulation of the tissues in an effort to restore them to normal resilience.

The choice of an antiseptic paint is a matter of individual preference, and has already been discussed in the chapter on postoperative procedure.

Compound Benzoin Tincture has the advantage of preventing the rapid "drying out" and subsequent hardening of the callus. There is no justification for the statement which is often made that the application of Friars' Balsam to an area of callus promotes healthy granulation. Granulation is the process by which a wound heals and has no relation at all to callus formation. Friars' Balsam may promote granulation of wounds but to use this expression when it is applied to callus is indefensible. Iodine Solution, Weak, and 0·5 per cent Hibitane in alcohol are also in common use as antiseptic paints.

As an alternative to an antiseptic paint, an astringent or a caustic may be used. It is difficult to classify these treatments under the headings, respectively, of *astringent* or *caustic*. Consider, for instance, the application of 40 per cent silver nitrate. As with most of the treatments noted below the efficacy of this method depends largely on the complete removal of the callus before the medicament is applied. The medicament has the apparent effect of reducing the rate of production and area of the callus. This cannot be classed properly either as a caustic or as an astringent action. It might be suggested that the silver nitrate acts by forming a tough coagulum on the surface of the epidermis which serves to reduce friction in the same way as the application of adhesive stockinette would do. It may also be the case that the application interferes in some way with the normal keratinization process. Medicaments which may be used following the removal of callus include 40 per cent solution of silver nitrate, 5 per cent solution of copper sulphate, 5 per cent solution of chromium trioxide and 5 per cent solution of trinitrophenol. Any of these may be applied to a large area after heavy callus has been removed or to a small area following the removal of a hard corn. They are also useful as application to interdigital soft corns, it being understood that the treatment of any local hyperidrosis is extremely important in dealing with such lesions.

A 1 per cent solution of crystal violet in spirit effects some quite remarkable results in the treatment of both hard and soft corns. It exerts an astringent action comparable to that of 40 per cent solution of silver nitrate, without producing a definite coagulum. The best results seem to be achieved when the solution is applied to a hard corn on the plantar surface. The nucleus must be removed as far as possible and the lesion completely saturated with the 1 per cent spirituous solution. It is worth spending two or three minutes to ensure that the growth is really saturated, using a fragment of cotton wool to rub the paint into the area. This preparation is also effective on interdigital corns when these are not excessively moist. Care must always be taken to ensure that the dye will not come off on patients' hose or, even more importantly, on their bed linen.

On an area of very moist callus the application of a paint of Liquefied Phenol or of 10 per cent solution of formalin is very effective. At each treatment a single coat of the medicament is painted on and allowed to dry before any dressings are applied. On an area of skin where the nutrition appears to be poor, or where there has been chilling, a thick paste of kaolin powder and water (*not Kaolin Poultice*) may be applied spread on lint. On a very inflamed callus, either a paint or a compress of Aluminium Acetate Solution may be applied or the kaolin paste technique may be employed. Another medicament which is useful in cases of heavy plantar callus is dichloroacetic acid. This acid is used at full strength and is painted on to the area after the removal of as much thickened stratum corneum as is possible. When the area has dried it may be covered with stockinette or adhesive padding, if so desired. The patient should return in two or three weeks time when a tough coagulum with loose and curled-over edges will have formed. Under the curled edges of the coagulum will be found healthy skin. The coagulum, following preliminary softening in a foot-bath, may often be peeled off with forceps. Repeated application of the acid will cause the callus gradually to diminish in size.

As an alternative after-dressing, an emollient may be used in order to soften and lubricate the skin. If the emollient is being applied by the chiropodist, for instance in a buffer pad, a rather heavy, stiff type of preparation is to be preferred, e.g. soft paraffin in which about 4 per cent of cetostearyl alcohol has been incorporated. On the other hand, if the patient is to apply the emollient daily at home a lighter, softer preparation may be employed. Hydrous Wool Fat Ointment is a favourite although there are some other preparations available which are rather less sticky and cosmetically more elegant. It should be made clear that a somewhat heavier preparation is required than the average hand creams obtainable from retail pharmacists. Whereas in the case of hairy skin the medicament will penetrate the invaginations in the skin, such as the sebaceous glands and the hair follicles, and so form a reserve, on glabrous skin the emollient must cling to the surface by virtue of its own viscosity.

Blank has shown by a simple experiment that stratum corneum becomes hard and brittle when it dries out. He has shown that it is impossible to replace the moisture which has been lost. The function of an emollient may in fact be to prevent too rapid loss of moisture from the horny layer, rather than the replacement of moisture which has been lost.

Corns and callus are frequently associated with a poor blood circulation. It will be noted that the word used is circulation and not supply. Local stasis of tissue fluid, the extreme example of which is the chilblain, does lead to the formation of callus. Lesions occurring over the site of chilblains are notoriously difficult to treat and it is particularly difficult to restore its natural elasticity and resilience to the skin. As an alternative to an astringent or an emollient, a rubefacient may be applied to an area of callus following the removal of the thickened stratum corneum. Iodine oil or Iodine Ointment Non-staining, either with or without methyl salicylate, may be used as the rubefacient. These preparations have an additional emollient action. When a compound containing methyl salicylate is used the part should not afterwards be covered as this tends to produce maceration of the area. Clove oil, turpentine oil and other rubefacients may also be used following the removal of plantar callus. What is much more effective than the application of a rubefacient by the chiropodist is the regular use of a scrubbing brush in the bath by the patient. A vigorous scrubbing of the skin with a fairly stiff nail brush will stimulate the skin and will do much to restore its normal elasticity and resilience. This form of treatment may be used not only for plantar callus but also for plantar and digital corns, with the additional feature that, in the case of corns, the tissues should also be kneaded and made mobile as far as possible. Restoration of the tissues' mobility is an important feature in the treatment of corns.

So far, the treatment of corns and callus has been discussed in general terms. Certain types of corn call for specific types of treatment. Thus the soft corn requires treatment of the hyperidrosis, with which it is often associated, while the local lesion itself calls for the use of a powerful astringent. Almost any of the astringents may be employed but it must be borne in mind that, if a strong (e.g. 2 per cent) solution of crystal violet in spirit is used, it will obliterate all the differences in tissue colour and will considerably increase the difficulties attendant on operating on an interdigital soft corn. On vascular corns pyrogallol (20 per cent ointment), silver nitrate (40 per cent solution), or ferric chloride (strong B.P.C. solution) are the medicaments of choice.

On a neurovascular corn ointments containing an analgesic, such as benzocaine 5 per cent, or orthocaine 5 per cent, produce relief of pain over a prolonged period of time.

It is re-iterated that if a corn is to be permanently eradicated very active treatment is required, especially in the initial cases. Very active treatment does not imply the use of strong drugs but rather the very frequent removal of the thickened skin. A corn or callus is too often allowed to re-establish itself before it is treated for a second time, so that the skin has no chance to return to normal. If the patient is seen two or three times a week and the corn or callus completely removed at each visit the skin will have a chance to regain its normal condition. The concept of treating a corn by curing it has not gained very much headway in the profession. Patients generally pay a fee for each visit and not for the treatment of a corn. If a corn is to be cured and not merely palliated the mechanical cause must be dealt with and the skin given every chance to recover. The idea is frequently mooted that the more a corn is cut, the more it will grow. But it must be pointed out firstly that the corn may itself be a source of irritation to the dermis, and secondly that the thickened stratum corneum of the corn may cause pressure keratinization in the deeper layers. This is a recognized defence mechanism against the invasion of skin epidermal growths into the deeper layers. Clearly it is important that the thickened stratum corneum should not be allowed to act in these ways and this is an additional reason why it must not be allowed to accumulate. Chiropodists must not rest content until corns and callus can be **cured**. To sum up, the main object in treating corns and callus is the restoration of the skin to its normal resilience and elasticity, bearing in mind that the word skin applies not solely to the epidermis but also to the dermis. It is highly probable that the formation of corns and callus is strongly influenced by the underlying dermis.

CHAPTER XII

THE TREATMENT OF WARTS

THE chiropodial technique for the treatment of plantar warts may be stated briefly as follows:

    (1) The removal with the scalpel of as much keratinized tissue as possible, without injury to the elongated papillae.

    (2) The destruction, by caustics or other means, of the remaining hyperkeratotic tissue and cells affected by the virus. Because the virus is an intracellular organism, this step includes *per se* the destruction of the virus itself.

Most operators develop a routine technique, the most popular of which is probably the use of salicylic ointment 60–70 per cent, either alone or with another acid. This treatment is applied on normally healthy patients with good circulations, where the condition of the skin surrounding the wart is good, where there is a reasonable amount of tissue between the wart and the underlying bone and where the patient can return at reasonable intervals of time. The provisos mentioned give an indication of the factors which influence the choice of treatments for a plantar wart. These factors are summarized below.

    (*a*) *The possibility of applying an ointment.* This depends on (i) the site of the wart, (ii) the condition of the skin surrounding the wart. Since warts on non-weightbearing parts tend to be more superficial than those on weightbearing surfaces they often respond quite readily to treatment with one of the liquid caustics or astringents. When the skin surrounding the part is macerated, a method of treatment which does not involve the use of adhesive padding must be employed. When maceration is due to the spreading of a previous application of salicylic acid, the skin may be hardened by the application of phenol or of 40 per cent solution of silver nitrate. The use of ointments is contra-indicated on very moist feet where the pad is likely to slip owing to the slippery nature of the skin.

    (*b*) *Size of growth.* Large growths lend themselves to treatment with ointments, small growths do not. If a large growth is surrounded by smaller growths the large growth may be treated with salicylic acid ointment and the smaller growths painted with trichloroacetic acid and Toughened Silver Nitrate.

    (*c*) *The necessity to keep the foot out of water.* If salicylic acid ointments or ointments of pyrogallol are used the foot must be kept out of water. If trichloroacetic acid with Toughened Silver Nitrate, phenol with nitric acid, or potassium hydroxide is used then the foot may be placed in water after the first twenty-four hours.

(d) *Where there is little adipose tissue between the growth and the bone.* Caustics which produce a breakdown are to be avoided. These are salicylic acid, monochloroacetic acid, pyrogallol and trichloroacetic acid when it is applied by rubbing the growth with a crystal of the acid.

(e) *On elderly patients.* Those having a poor circulation and those with diabetes should have their warts treated with the milder caustics in preference to those mentioned in (d) above.

(f) *The availability of the patient.* If salicylic, pyrogallol, monochloroacetic acid or carbon dioxide snow is used it is essential that the patient should return within the stipulated period, generally fourteen days, and it is desirable that he should be able to contact the practitioner at any time during the period of treatment. If silver nitrate or one of the other astringents is used, or if silver nitrate with trichloroacetic acid is used, the return period is less important and, although it is desirable that patients should return in 7–14 days, if they are prevented from doing so, no serious harm will result. If nitric acid and phenol or potassium hydroxide is used, each treatment is completed during the time the patient is in the surgery. These treatments are useful when the patient can report for treatment only at irregular intervals. If a patient who is being treated with salicylic acid has to break a course of treatments, for instance, to go on holiday, the last application of salicylic acid should be made fourteen days before the patient's final visit prior to the break in treatment. The patient should return seven days before the final treatment, and both this penultimate treatment and the final one should be applications of Toughened Silver Nitrate. Normal treatment may then be resumed when the patient returns from holiday. When rapid results are required carbon dioxide snow or potassium hydroxide should be used, but both these techniques may cause pain. They should not be used on young children but may be indicated for active, healthy patients where there is a reasonable amount of tissue between the lesion and underlying bone.

Obstinate Growths which do not Respond to Routine Treatment

A growth which has been unsuccessfully treated with X-ray is often very difficult to remove and the patient should be warned that treatment may be prolonged. In the early stages, the size of the growth may be reduced by using silver nitrate and trichloroacetic acid and the final fragments may be treated with pyrogallol or potassium hydroxide. The use either of salicylic acid or of silver nitrate by itself are to be avoided in this type of growth.

Where a growth does not respond to one form of treatment it may do so to another, and any one form of treatment should not be continued too long. Very often an application of potassium hydroxide will help to move an obstinate growth and, if such a growth is a shallow one, a useful alternative is nitric acid and phenol. If a series of treatments is very prolonged it is often advisable to give the patient a complete rest from it for a month or six weeks, padding the foot to give comfort, if necessary. Another type of obstinate growth is one which appears on the site of a breakdown from a previous treatment. It is important in such a case to be sure that the lesion is a wart and not a scar from a healed ulcer.

Very often some form of mechanical irritation is associated with obstinate growths. For example, a deep growth may occur between or over the metatarsal heads. The reason for lack of response to treatment is the continued mechanical irritation. The answer to this type of case is to pad the lesion exactly as if it were a hard corn, e.g. in a case such as that quoted above, a metatarsal shaft or prop should be incorporated in the padding. Sometimes very heavy padding is required but generally this may be discontinued as soon as the wart is cleared.

A wart is clear when all the affected cells have been destroyed and the tissues have returned to their normal condition. The point at which to cease treatment, short of producing a breakdown of tissue, is a matter learned by experience but, as a guide, it may be said that a wart may be considered clear when the skin presents an unbroken appearance and there is no pain on side pressure.

A Summary of the More Common Forms of Wart Treatment

Salicylic Acid Ointment, 60–70 per cent (page 206)
Indications: Routine treatment, when it is possible to apply an acid ointment by means of a pad. The foot must be kept out of water.

Contra-indications: When a breakdown of tissue is to be avoided, or on a very moist foot.

Return Period: From 5–21 days. Seven days is the usual interval although a better result with less maceration of surrounding skin may be obtained with a fourteen-day interval.

See also *para*-hydroxybenzoic acid (page 208).

Salicylic Acid Ointment with Monochloroacetic Acid (page 193)

Indications: On larger growths on a healthy patient where there is sufficient adipose tissue underlying the wart. The foot must be kept out of water.

Contra-indications: When breakdown is to be avoided and when the patient cannot easily contact the chiropodist.

Return period: 5–7 days.

25 per cent Salicylic Acid and 25 per cent Lactic Acid Ointment

Indications: When a milder ointment treatment is required, e.g. for young children.

Contra-indications: As for salicylic acid.

Return period: 7–14 days.

Monochloroacetic Acid (page 193)

Indications: Cases in which an ointment cannot be applied, or as an alternative to salicylic acid on normal cases.

Contra-indications: When a breakdown is to be avoided.

Return period: 3–14 days, generally 7 days.

Trichloroacetic Acid with or without Toughened Silver Nitrate (page 219)

Indications: Shallow growths, mosaic warts and warts occurring on such sites as the nail grooves and interdigital clefts. The foot need not be kept out of water after the first 24 hours.

Contra-indications: Deep growths, or when rapid results are required.

Return period: Minimum 4 days, optimum 7–10 days.

Nitric Acid and Phenol (page 194)

Indications: Shallow multiple growths and as an alternative treatment on obstinate growths. The foot need not be kept out of water.

Contra-indications: Nervous patients.

Return period: 3–4 days, may be longer.

Phenol (page 198)

Indications: On the moist feet and in cases where the skin has been badly macerated by salicylic acid.

Contra-indications: Young children, very elderly patients or diabetic patients, or in cases of circulatory insufficiency.

Return period: 3–4 days, may be longer.

Potassium Hydroxide (page 201)

Indications: When rapid results are required or on obstinate growths where treatment with acids has failed.

Contra-indications: When the patient has a poor circulation or is in poor general health, or on very shallow growths.

Return period: Action is immediate.

Pyrogallol (page 203)

Indications: Very vascular or painful growths. As an alternative to salicylic acid when the tissues are badly macerated.

Return period: 5–14 days, generally 7 days.

Contra-indications: In cases where the skin is either very moist or very dry, with elderly or diabetic cases, and where the circulation or underlying soft tissue is inadequate.

Carbon Dioxide Snow (page 159)

Indications: Obstinate growths or when quick results are required.

Contra-indications: When a breakdown is to be avoided.

Return period: 5–10 days according to the technique used.

Podophyllum Resin (10 per cent in spirit) (page 200)

Indications: For home treatment or when a very mild treatment is required.

The Astringents

Silver Nitrate (page 210), Formalin (page 174), Alum (page 144), 25 per cent Chromium Trioxide Solution, Copper Sulphate (page 167).

Indications: For shallow growths occurring on non-weightbearing areas. For the clearing of final fragments (Toughened Silver Nitrate).

Contra-indications: The Silver Nitrate Stick should not be used alone for more than two consecutive treatments without an alternative treatment being tried.

Occlusion

Covering a wart with Elastoplast or, better, waterproof strapping, will sometimes produce effective maceration. This form of treatment is uncertain but works rapidly in some cases.

Indications: Where other forms of treatment are contra-indicated, on large groups of warts or mosaic warts.

Return period: 7–14 days, may be longer.

The Treatment of Ulcers Produced by the Action of Acids

When a slough or breakdown is produced by the action of an acid the resulting ulcer will generally heal very rapidly provided it is not allowed to become wet and soggy. If it does become soggy, healing will be slow and there will be a tendency for the wart to re-establish itself. Because of this Proflavine and Aminacrine Cream and similar preparations are contra-indicated. An application of silver nitrate 10 per cent solution, or other astringent of comparable strength, will generally produce a good result. Because of the acid the ulcer will be sterile and generally an astringent plus an occlusive, but not air-tight dressing, is sufficient protection. If an antiseptic is required one of the amino-acridines in spirit or a water-soluble jelly base, "Viacu-tan" or "Ponoxylan Gel" may be used. Also 10 per cent Ichthammol in glycerine may be used. The ulcer should heal in two or three days.

NOTE

Caustic ointments may be applied to localized lesions such as warts or deep corns and the chief problem is to confine the acid to the area to be treated. The ointment is almost invariably applied by means of an aperture pad, the aperture being slightly larger in size than the lesion, so that it will serve both as a container for the caustic ointment and as a protective dressing. Compound Benzoin Tinc-ture is painted on to the surrounding skin right up to the edge of the lesion. A piece of stockinette or strapping, having a hole in it slightly smaller than the lesion, is then placed over the latter. When the pad has been fixed in position the pad cavity is filled with the appropriate ointment and sealed by covering with adhesive strapping. When the patient returns it will be found invariably that the area which has been macerated by the acid coincides *with the aperture cut in the pad.* It will be seen that some protection has been afforded by the Compound Benzoin Tinc-ture and the stockinette or strapping, but this protection is by no means complete. Instead of the Compound Benzoin Tincture a layer of flexible collodion or of silver nitrate solution may be painted on to the skin surrounding the lesion and allowed to dry. A solution of silver nitrate 10 per cent is used for this purpose. Neither of these methods affords complete protection. It must be remembered that a caustic ointment acts in all directions and not only vertically to the surface of the epidermis. It is of importance that the pad containing the ointment should be very firmly fixed to the skin because, if it were to slip, it would mean that the ointment was being applied to a healthy area of skin. Absorption of the ointment by the material of the pad may be minimized by painting the walls of the aperture with either Compound Benzoin Tincture or with flexible collodion. An alternative method of applying a caustic ointment is to smear a small quantity on to the lesion and, if possible, to rub it into the latter with a small flexible spatula, and then to cover it with *waterproof* strapping. This method gives as effective a result as using larger quantities of ointment in an aperture pad, and there is very little tendency for the ointment to spread because the amount used is small.

With the advent of new apparatus and of the use of local analgesics two major physical methods of destroying wart tissue have been added to the chiropodist's armarmentarium—fulguration, electro-dessication, and the use of liquid nitrous oxide which gives lower temperatures than carbon dioxide snow. Neither treat-ment has the disadvantages associated with the use of caustic ointments which are difficult to use on certain sites and are unsuitable for use in cases of multiple warts. After a brief initial period the foot need not be kept out of water. These techniques can be very effective in the hands of experienced operators. The apparatus is fairly expensive but, even before they have the status of routine treat-ments, their use may be indicated in lieu of potassium hydroxide, nitric acid and silver nitrate with trichloroacetic acid. Their action is probably more easily con-trolled than that of salicylic acid used in conjunction with monchloro–acetic acid.

CHAPTER XIII

THE TREATMENT OF HYPERIDROSIS, BROMIDROSIS AND ANHIDROSIS

HYPERIDROSIS or Hyperhidrosis means excessive sweating; Bromidrosis means excessive sweating accompanied by an offensive odour; Anhidrosis means diminution of sweating. These are the dictionary definitions. Hyperidrosis is recognized by dampness of the skin, maceration and, in some cases, inflammation and blistering. There is little difficulty in recognizing a hyperidrotic skin. A little thought will show, however, that in cases labelled respectively, hyperidrosis or anhidrosis, there is no evidence of any excessive or diminished sweating *except the condition of the skin*. Maceration of the skin can be produced quite easily by covering it with waterproof plaster and preventing the evaporation of the sweat. It must be clearly understood that in most cases referred to as hyperidrosis or anhidrosis a condition of the skin is meant and this may or may not be related to the amount of sweat secreted by the sweat glands. The condition we know as hyperidrosis may be produced as easily by non-evaporation of sweat, or by the inability of the skin to tolerate sweat, as by excessive sweating.

The mechanisms which control the amount of secretion of the sweat glands in the palms of the hands and the soles of the feet are quite different from that controlling sweating of the rest of the body's surface. Insensible perspiration is moisture which discharges through the skin as water vapour; sweating, that is secretion from the sweat glands, only takes place on exercise or when the temperature of the body's environment is raised. On the palms and soles the sweat glands secrete all the time. Sweating of the general body surface, excluding the palms and the soles, is part of the mechanism for maintaining the body at a steady temperature and is therefore under thermal control. The function of the sweat is to cause the body to lose heat by the evaporation of moisture from the surface of the skin. The function of the sweat on the palms and soles is different. There are no sebaceous glands in the skin in these areas and in them the sweat performs an important function in keeping the skin moist and therefore supple. Sweating of the palms and soles is only slightly increased by a rise in temperature but it is easily increased by mental

110

or sensory stimuli. Mental or emotional stress is a common cause of hyperidrosis of the feet, as is a fatigued or strained foot. In exercise both thermal and mental factors are involved and sweating will take place over the whole of the body surface. Because sweating of the palms and soles has a different function from sweating over the rest of the body surface, the stimulus which produces it is different. It may not be appreciated that a local hyperidrosis may be associated with a mechanical stress, which may determine the site at which the maceration due to excess sweating manifests itself. Maceration of a localized area of skin may be due to a hyperidrosis associated with mechanical trauma, such as friction over that particular area: or it may be that the friction causes a diminution of the skin's resistance to the macerating effect of the sweat.

In bromidrosis the foul odour is due to the breakdown products of the sweat. This breakdown may be due to bacterial activity but there is very little accurate information on this point. Breakdown may also occur when evaporation of the sweat is slow and it remains on the skin long enough for breakdown to take place. This is one of the reasons why the establishment of evaporation is so important in the management of such cases.

It has been pointed out above that the function of the sweat on the palms of the hands and the soles of the feet is to keep the thick epidermis of these areas moist and therefore supple. Anhidrosis, which would probably be better termed *hypohidrosis*, leads to a dryness of the skin with loss of elasticity, which may cause fissuring, and to hardness of the skin which means that the rate of desquamation from the surface of the epidermis is diminished and the stratum corneum becomes thickened.

It must be stressed that the chiropodist is interested in the effect of the disorders of the sweat glands on the skin. Hyperidrosis and bromidrosis result in maceration and soreness and, in severe cases, blistering may occur. Maceration of the skin leads to weakness and loss of elasticity which may result in fissuring and also to a diminution of the skin's resistance to bacterial and fungal infections. Anhidrosis results in a hardening and thickening of the stratum corneum which may lead to brittleness and loss of elasticity which, again, may result in fissuring.

The Treatment of the Skin Conditions associated with Hyperidrosis and Bromidrosis

The first step in the treatment of the skin conditions associated with hyperidrosis is to bring about, wherever possible, a reduction in the amount of sweat secreted by the sweat glands. The first line of approach is generally to relieve strain and congestion in the foot. The strain may be treated by mechanical means or by exercises and physical methods. Since the sweating of the palms and soles is not brought about by thermal stimulation, contrast foot-baths, which are frequently so successful in the treatment of hyperidrosis, probably alleviate the condition by virtue of their effect in relieving strain and congestion in the feet. The drying of the feet with a rough towel after bathing has a similar effect. Hyperidrosis is frequently the result of of emotional disturbances and once the condition has become established it, in turn, produces a feeling of guilt so that a vicious circle is set up. The breaking of this circle calls for tact and enthusiasm on the part of the chiropodist and it is extremely important that the patient should feel that the chiropodist is interested in his condition and has the ability to cure him; treatment, unless the patient is so convinced, is useless. This is important in the whole patient-chiropodist relationship but it is never so important as in the treatment of hyperidrosis and bromidrosis, regarding which it is all too easy to give a string of rather weary routine instructions regarding foot hygiene. Need it be added that the chiropodist, even involuntarily, must never betray any aversion to the patient with the hyperidrotic or bromidrotic foot! In severe cases reference to the physician or surgeon may be necessary.

Apart from steps to reduce the flow of sweat, the treatment of skin conditions associated with hyperidrosis is, in general, directed to:

1. Ensuring that the sweat does not accumulate, and is in contact with the skin for the shortest possible time.

2. Increasing the skin's resistance to the action of the sweat.

3. The use of antiseptics and fungicides to counteract the loss of the skin's natural resistance to infection.

The steps taken to ensure that the sweat does not accumulate may be summed up under three general headings:

1. *Personal hygiene.* This involves the regular washing of the feet and their careful drying after washing. The use of a rough towel in drying, to reduce congestion, has already been mentioned.

2. *Aeration.* In order that evaporation from the skin may take place there must be a flow of air round the skin. If the air over the skin becomes saturated with water vapour no evaporation can take place. In summer it may be convenient for the patient to go without socks or stockings and to wear sandals. It is very important that ordinary shoes should not be worn when socks or stockings have

been discarded. Apart from the fact that the shoes may irritate the tender skin, there will be very little increase in the amount of evaporation which takes place and also it is difficult to dry the inside of ordinary footwear. In all cases of patients who suffer from hyperidrosis it is important that the footwear should not be made of impermeable materials such as rubber, certain plastics, etc. It is also highly desirable that the patient should not wear the same pair of shoes on consecutive days. One of the finest treatments for patients suffering from hyperidrosis is for them to sit in the fresh air with their feet exposed to the sun.

3. *Absorbents*. Work carried out by the Shoes and Allied Trades Research Association has shown that a substantial amount of sweat, possibly more than half the total produced, is absorbed by the footwear, particularly the insoles and uppers. The experiments were conducted on men wearing shoes made of conventional materials. The results showed some variation, but established quite clearly that footwear plays an important role in sweat absorbtion. Clearly, drying-out of shoes is important especially if they are to be worn next day. It is also clearly desirable that the materials used in shoe manufacture should have a high water-vapour permeability, thus allowing as much evaporation of sweat as possible, so reducing the amount to be absorbed by the footwear. It is also suggested that detachable insocks, which can be removed from the shoe for drying-out, are desirable.

Hosiery is also an important absorbent and in addition the shed skin cells and debris will collect in the hose. It is important that the patient should wear hosiery that is capable of taking up moisture. All wool or a wool synthetic mixture is satisfactory, but spun nylon, or similar synthetic material which resembles wool in appearance and absorbative properties, is perhaps the best material for hose for a hyperidrotic patient. Spun nylon washes well, dries quickly and does not shrink or felt. The hose need not be of a heavy weave, in fact lightly woven socks are to be preferred. It is important that the patient should realize that the absorbative capacity of the material is limited so that frequent changes of hose are necessary and it is elementary common sense that the hose must be washed before being used again, and not merely dried. Foot-powders are not significant as absorbents. Too little is applied to absorb more than a minute fraction of the sweat. But, since sweating tends to increase the coefficient of friction of the skin, the lubricating qualities of foot-powders are important in maintaining foot comfort.

The use of astringents in the treatment of skin conditions due to hyperidrosis has, empirically, been proved to be successful. Their mode of action is not precisely known. It has been suggested that (*a*) they may exert some direct action on the sweat glands themselves which, from an anatomical point of view alone, seems unlikely, or (*b*) they may act by blocking the sweat glands through mechanical closure at the orifices, which again seems improbable. In the writer's opinion, it is more likely that they act upon the skin cells and so alter them that they are made more resistant to the action of the sweat. An example of this is provided by formalin which, it is suggested, acts by preventing maceration of the skin rather than by reducing the amount of sweat secreted. The astringent may be applied as a powder or lotion, or in the form of a foot-bath. The most common skin conditions resulting from excessive sweating are maceration, which is sometimes accompanied by a marked degree of inflammation due to irritation of the skin through the presence of accumulated sweat, fissuring and, in severe cases, blistering of the skin. The effect of hyperidrosis on the skin is also to lower its resistance to infection by bacterial, and especially by fungal, organisms. It is therefore an advantage to incorporate a fungicide or an antiseptic in some stage of the treatment.

In general the treatment of skin conditions associated with hyperidrosis and bromidrosis consists of the prescription of a routine for the regular washing of the feet, followed by careful drying with a rough towel, if the skin will tolerate this; the regular changing of the hose and the drying of shoes between wearing. The washing of the feet may be followed by a foot-bath or the application of a lotion followed by the use of a dusting powder.

Suitable medicaments for use in cases of hyperidrosis and bromidrosis are mentioned below:

For use in the surgery.

Compound Benzoin Tincture, applied to mild interdigital maceration.

Chromium trioxide, a 5 per cent aqueous solution, applied once a week.

Formalin, a 10 per cent aqueous solution, painted on to the skin and allowed to dry. This is a suitable application for severe cases and may be repeated at fortnightly intervals.

Silver nitrate as an aqueous solution up to 10 per cent strength according to the severity of the case. An alternative method is to paint the macerated skin with a 5 per cent solution of silver nitrate followed by a paint of saline solution. Silver chloride is formed and is allowed to dry on the skin.

Trinitrophenol as a 5 per cent aqueous solution.

The lotions listed above have the advantage of being antiseptic and fungicidal as well as astringent.

For daily use by the patient at home.

Alcohol, as Surgical Spirit.

Aluminium acetate, as Aluminium Acetate Solution B.P.C. diluted one part to three parts of water. This is particularly useful where maceration is accompanied by inflammation.

Calamine, as Calamine Lotion B.P.

Copper sulphate, a 1 per cent aqueous solution.

Hamamelis, as Hamamelis Water B.P.C., when there is marked inflammation.

Salicylic acid, 3 per cent solution in spirit.

Foot-baths for home use (quantities given are for half a gallon [2½ litres] of water). Contrast foot-baths in plain water. Two bowls are used, one containing warm water (46° C. [115° F.]) and the other water from the cold tap. The feet are placed first in the warm water for about one minute and then in the cold water for 10–15 seconds and the process is repeated three or four times, ending with the feet in warm water.

Saline: 2–3 tablespoonfuls of common salt or "Tidman's Sea Salt".

Magnesium sulphate: 2 tablespoonfuls.

Potassium permanganate: sufficient crystals to cover the end of a matchstick. The final solution should be pinkish rather than purple in colour.

Formalin: 30 ml. of 10 per cent solution or 4 ml. (one teaspoonful) of 40 per cent solution.

Solution of Chloroxylenol B.P.: 45 ml.

Cresol with Soap Solution B.P.: 30 ml.

Sodium polymetaphosphate: 2–3 tablespoonfuls.

(*For home reckoning one tablespoonful is roughly 15 ml.*)

Dusting-powders. The dusting-powders used for hyperidrosis will generally have a base such as kaolin, talc, zinc oxide, bismuth carbonate, etc. In addition to the base, an astringent such as salicylic acid, tannic acid, alum, or sodium polymetaphosphate and an antiseptic or fungicide such as boric acid, salicylic acid, camphor, menthol, sulphur, phenyl mercuric nitrate or undecenoic acid may be incorporated in the dusting-powder. One of the advantages of using dusting-powders in the treatment of hyperidrosis and bromidrosis is that they may include a number of ingredients giving a wide range of action.

Apart from the value of their active ingredients, dusting-powders act as lubricants, offsetting the increase in the coefficient of friction of the skin associated with excess sweating.

The official dusting-powders include:

Chlorphenesin Dusting-powder B.P.C. (chlorphenesin 1, starch 56, zinc oxide 25, talc 18).

Hexachlorophane Dusting-powder B.P.C. (hexachlorophane 0·3, zinc oxide 3, absorbable dusting-powder 96·7).

Talc Dusting-powder B.P.C. (talc 90, starch 10).

Zinc and Salicylic Acid Dusting-powder B.P.C. (salicylic acid 5, zinc oxide 20, starch 75).

Zinc, Starch and Talc Dusting-powder B.P.C. (zinc oxide 25, starch 25, talc 50).

Zinc Undecenoate Dusting-powder B.P.C. (starch 50, zinc undecenoate 10, undecenoic acid 2, kaolin 38).

There are also many excellent proprietary foot-powders available, some of which are listed on page 13.

In some cases of severe hyperidrosis blistering of the skin may occur. These blisters are somewhat difficult to dress and to treat as they are generally very sore. It is desirable, if possible, to avoid opening the blister. Iodine Solution, Weak B.P., may be painted on to encourage absorption of the fluid, or a paint consisting of equal parts of Compound Benzoin Tincture and Iodine Solution, Strong B.P., may be used. Alternatively, Compound Benzoin Tincture or Flexible Collodion may be used as an antiseptic and protective paint. If the blister has burst or has been opened, a solution of aminacrine in spirit may be employed as an antiseptic dressing. These treatments may be followed by the use of an astringent powder to treat the generalized hyperidrosis. When the blisters have healed, steps should be taken to prevent irritation of the particular area involved and also to harden the skin in order to prevent their recurrence.

Owing to the loss of the skin's elasticity, fissuring may accompany hyperidrosis. Generally this occurs between the toes and it may be associated with a mycotic infection. The loss of skin elasticity may be due either to the hyperidrosis or to the mycotic infection. The treatment of these fissures consists of the application of an astringent and antiseptic or fungicidal paint. Compound Benzoin Tincture is often sufficiently active to promote their healing if, at the same time, steps are taken to reduce the general hyperidrosis. Salicylic acid 3 per cent may be incorporated in the Compound Benzoin Tincture. Other astringent paints which may be used are 5 per cent salicylic acid in spirit, 5 per cent silver nitrate in distilled water or spirit, and 1–2 per cent crystal violet in spirit. A 1–500 solution of phenyl mercuric nitrate in isopropyl alcohol is a useful astringent, fungicide and antiseptic. This may be applied to gauze or lint, the saturated dressing being left between the toes for 5 or 10 minutes; in some cases gauze dressings may be left *in situ* for several days.

The Treatment of Skin Conditions associated with Anhidrosis

Although it is clear that a deficiency in the secretion of the sweat glands causes dryness and lack of skin elasticity, it is by no means certain that dryness of the skin is caused always by lack of activity of the sweat glands. It should be understood that this section deals with general dryness of the skin and is not confined solely to conditions associated with defective sweat secretion. Unfortunately, there is little that can be done to stimulate permanently the activity of the sweat glands and, generally, only local treatment is possible.

Much of the treatment of skin dryness has been discussed in the chapter on the treatment of corns and callus and only a brief recapitulation of the principles of treatment will be given here.

If there is gross thickening of stratum corneum the keratinized tissues may be softened by the use of salicylic acid, it being remembered that salicylic acid only softens and does not remove the hardened tissues. As an alternative potassium hydroxide may be used in the form of crude soft soap. Simple dryness or flaking of the skin may be treated by the application either of an emollient ointment which is fatty or greasy in nature, or of a cream or ointment containing a high proportion of water. Suitable preparations include:

Parenol B.P.C. 1949 (white soft paraffin 65, wool fat 15, and water 20).

Simple Ointment B.P. (soft paraffin 85, wool fat 5, hard paraffin 5, cetostearyl alcohol 5).

Emulsifying Ointment B.P. (emulsifying wax 30, white soft paraffin 50, liquid paraffin 20).

Aqueous Cream B.P. consists of 30 per cent of Emulsifying Ointment, 0·1 per cent chlorocresol with distilled water to 100 per cent.

Hydrous Wool Fat Ointment B.P.C. (Lanolin Ointment) (equal parts of hydrous wool fat and yellow soft paraffin).

Preparations containing almond oil, cod-liver oil, arachis oil or olive oil are preferred by some operators but these are generally very greasy.

Frequent gentle scrubbing with a soft nail brush using soap and water, helps to stimulate the skin and to increase its elasticity and resilience. Elderly patients tend to suffer from dryness of the skin associated with poor peripheral blood supply. If it is possible for the patient to carry out the scrubbing routine this will help considerably, but very often it is beyond his power to do this. Irritant drugs are contra-indicated because of the skin's poor response, and drugs such as salicylic acid, and especially silver nitrate, are to be avoided. Wherever the skin is dry, silver nitrate must be used with great caution since on a normal skin its action is modified considerably by the sodium chloride present in the skin. Aqueous Cream B.P. is one of the most satisfactory emollients for use by elderly patients.

With the dryness and loss of elasticity of the skin, fissuring may occur where the skin is subjected to tension. The common sites are between the toes and round the heels. The technique for dealing with such fissures is to remove any thickened stratum corneum from the edges of the lesion and to apply an emollient and/or healing preparation such as Compound Benzoin Tincture, Proflavine or Aminacrine Cream or Ichthammol Glycerin. Salicylic Acid Collodion may be used in order to soften the hard edges of the fissures and this may be followed by a paint of from 5 to 25 per cent solution of silver nitrate if it is necessary to counteract excessive softening. Ointments containing ichthammol or Peru Balsam are also useful for treating these lesions.

CHAPTER XIV

THE TREATMENT OF FUNGAL INFECTION OF THE SKIN AND NAILS

DERMATOMYCOSIS is due to infection of the skin by one of the higher fungi, the common genera being *Trichophyton*, *Epidermophyton* and *Candida*. The identification of the infecting species is a job for an expert mycologist, but a chiropodist who possesses a microscope can frequently establish the fact that fungal infection has occurred by identifying mycelia in epithetial debris. The reader is referred to a larger work on dermatology for the technique of taking and preparing scrapings for microscopic examination. Some general observations can be made, which apply equally to taking scrapings which are to be sent to a mycologist. Obviously scrapings should be taken before any medication is begun. If, however, fungicides have been used these should be discontinued for at least one week, and preferably longer, before the samples of skin are taken. Samples of skin stained with dyes are useless for the purpose of examination. It is, for reasons which are not apparent, very difficult to culture fungi from nail clippings or scrapings. It is therefore of value to submit scrapings from skin adjacent to the nail whether or not this is exhibiting a clinical fungal infection. The specimens from nail and adjacent skin should be submitted in separate envelopes to the laboratory as different techniques will be used to examine them. The amount of material made available to the laboratory should be as large as possible. It is a common finding in laboratories that interdigital scrapings from the feet consist entirely of talc powder. The interdigital spaces should be washed well with normal saline solution (*not* with pre-operative detergent which may have fungicidal properties) before the scrapings are taken.

A wide range of drugs are effective against pathogenic fungi, including the following:

Benzoic Acid as Compound Benzoic Acid Ointment.
Borotannic Complex as "Medistan" or "Phytex".
Camphor as Camphor Oil.
Chlorbutol as "Mycozol".
Chlorphenesin as "Mycil".
Copper Sulphate as Copper and Zinc Sulphates Lotion.

TC–E

119

Crystal Violet as Compound Crystal Violet Paint.

Diamethazole as "Asterol".

Dibromopropamide Isethionate as a 0·15 per cent Cream.

Domiphen Bromide as a 0·5 per cent solution in 70 per cent Isopropyl Alcohol.

Fenticlor as "S7".

Halethazole as "Episol".

Hydrargaphen as "Penotrane".

Iodine as a Solution, weak or strong.

Magenta as Magenta Paint.

Pecilocin, an antibiotic (see page 150), as "Variotin".

Peru Balsam as 12·5 per cent Ointment.

Phenylmercuric Acetate as "Phytodermine Cream".

Phenylmercuric Nitrate as a Solution, Cream or Dusting-powder.

Potassium Hydroxyquinoline Sulphate as 1:2,000 solution.

Potassium Permanganate as a Solution or Foot-bath.

Propionic Acid as Ointment (2·5–3·5 per cent) or Dusting-powder (0·25 per cent).

Salicylic Acid as Ointment (up to 10 per cent), Alcoholic Solution (3–5 per cent), Dusting-powder (5 per cent), or with Compound Benzoin Tincture (5 per cent) or Collodion (12 per cent).

Sodium Polymetaphosphate as a Dusting-powder (5 per cent).

Thiomersal as "Merthiolate" or "Metaphen".

Tolnaftate as "Tineaderm".

Undecenoic Acid and Zinc Undecenoate as Ointment or Dusting-powder or as "Mycota", "Tineafax", "Amoxal", "Episol" or "Phytocil".

The management of fungal infections calls for much patience on the part of both operator and patient. It is generally undesirable, while the fungus is clinically active, to persist with one line of treatment over long periods. A change in treatment will often bring about an improvement in the condition. When the clinical symptoms have been relieved it is important to continue with local treatment for a considerable period of time. A fungicidal dusting-powder is useful for this purpose. Attention must be paid to potential foci of infection, especially the nails. Infected shoes and stockings should be treated in order to prevent re-infection from these sources. The hose should be boiled for 10 minutes prior to inclusion in the family wash. This rules out the use of woollen hosiery which cannot be boiled. Skin squames containing viable fungi have been recovered after as many as two hundred consecutive washings using soaps and various fungicides.

Shoes may be treated with acetaldehyde vapour using the same method as for formalin vapour described on page 175.

Infection is spread by infected skin squames. These adhere very firmly by atmospheric pressure to smooth surfaces. It is therefore important that slipper-baths, foot-baths and shower cubicles be vigorously scrubbed down with copious running water after each use by members of a community suffering from fungal infection of the feet. It is a wise precaution to use disposable paper coverings on bath mats, and to use paper towels to dry the feet. Both sets of paper should be burned after use.

The treatment of dermatomycosis may be related to the signs and symptoms produced and it is convenient to divide up the common manifestations of mycotic infection thus:

(a) Vesicular eruptions.
(b) Chronic intertrigo.
(c) Hyperkeratotic or eczematoid lesions.
(d) Pyodermic conditions due to secondary infection with bacteria.
(e) "id" or "ide" conditions.

The vesicular stage of mycotic infection may present in a number of different ways. There may be small discrete vesicles, which may coalesce to give a "sago-skin" appearance, or there may be large lesions having an actively inflamed edge. In most cases the fungus is in the superficial layers of the skin and fungicidal lotions, paints and non-greasy ointments are indicated. If the vesicular stage is at all severe it should be referred at once to a dermatologist.

Intertrigo occurs where two skin surfaces are in apposition, e.g. the interdigital clefts, and the manifestations are maceration and itching, with fissuring in some cases. Chronic intertrigo is by no means always due to fungal infection but the possibility must be borne in mind. Treatment of any accompanying hyperidrotic condition must be instituted. Local treatment consists of preparations which are both fungicidal and astringent: fungicidal ointments may also be used. In the first category, Compound Benzoin Tincture with 5 per cent of salicylic acid added, 3–5 per cent of salicylic acid in spirit, Magenta Paint, and phenylmercuric nitrate 1 in 500 of isopropyl alcohol, are favourite remedies. With the exception of Magenta Paint, these may be applied daily by the patient at home. The regular use of a fungicidal dusting-powder is a valuable auxiliary to the paint. Compound Benzoic Acid Ointment may be used but it must be remembered that this ointment is keratolytic and may cause considerable soreness if applied between the toes. Ointments containing the inorganic salts of mercury are also useful, but more modern practice calls for those containing phenylmercuric nitrate or acetate, undecenoic acid or its salts, propionic acid, caprylic acid or chlorophenesin. It is preferable to use ointments which are prepared in a non-greasy base.

Chronic hyperkeratotic or eczematoid lesions call for medicaments which are capable of penetrating the horny layer of the skin and so reaching the infected tissue. Removal of a thickened stratum corneum with the knife or a Moore's disc should be carried out as far as possible before applying the fungicide. Salicylic Acid Collodion may be painted on and left for 14 days in order to soften the hardened tissues and facilitate its removal with the scalpel.

Whitfield's Ointment is a well-tested remedy but one which, if applied properly, may destroy the epidermis and cause soreness. Magenta Paint or paints containing crystal violet or thymol are also useful. Strong Solution of Iodine is an alternative medicament.

Pyodermic Conditions due to Secondary Infections

These will frequently require to be referred to a dermatologist. In mild cases the application of antiseptic lotions such as 1:1,000 solution of phenylmercuric nitrate (which is both antiseptic and fungicidal), 1:1,000 solution of mercuric chloride, 1:1,000 solution of aminacrine in spirit or in distilled water may be sufficient. Calamine Lotion with Coal Tar is an alternative. These lotions should be applied as gauze soaks bandaged into position. If the condition does not respond rapidly the case should be referred to a dermatologist.

"Id" Conditions

These are secondary eruptions occurring at a distance from the site of infection, for example on the hands of a patient suffering from *tinea pedis*. They may occur on the feet. They contain no viable fungi and are best referred to a dermatologist.

THE TREATMENT OF ONYCHOMYCOSIS

The treatment of fungal infection of the nail calls for active and prolonged treatment. It is a very difficult condition to cure but it is important that it should be treated because otherwise the nails may form a focus leading to skin infection. The method of treatment is to remove as much as possible of the infected nail, also the debris which accumulates under the nail plate. Penetrating fungicides are applied following removal of the infected material.

One of the most effective paints is Iodine Solution, Strong. A 1 per cent spirituous solution of crystal violet may be applied and phenol-camphor mixtures are effective in some cases. The use of Borotannic complex has proved effective in many cases. Salicylic Acid Collodion may be painted on to the affected tissues with a view to preparing them for the subsequent action of a fungicide and the salicylic acid itself is fungicidal. Generally the ointments and creams are not notably effective but may be used as alternative treatments. Paste of Bismuth Subnitrate and Iodoform may be rubbed into an infected nail, which should be left uncovered.[1] It has been said that Magenta Paint does not give good results in the treatment of onychomycosis. It must be realized that to clear up a case of onychomycosis entirely will take at least as long as it takes for a completely new nail to form, that is, from 6 to 9 months, and it is well that both patient and operator should understand this. Undoubtedly the most important feature of treatment is the regular and complete removal of infected nail, a procedure a chiropodist is well equipped to carry out.

It is interesting that the systemic use of the antibiotic, Griseofulvin, produces fair results in cases of onychomycosis of the fingernails but very poor results in onychomycosis of toe nails.

[1] This is best used in conjunction with an Iodine Solution.

CHAPTER XV

THE TREATMENT OF PLASTER DERMATITIS

Plaster dermatitis is an inflammation of the skin which results from the application of adhesive plaster. The manifestations may be erythema, a papular rash, or a vesicular rash which may become secondarily infected to produce pustules or eczematous skin lesions. It is also thought that, in some instances, fungal infection latent in the skin may be exacerbated by the application of adhesive plasters. The plaster rash may be caused by chemical irritation from the ingredients of the adhesive mass; by mechanical irritation due to suction, or to friction between the pad and the skin; by the interference with the normal functions of the skin, or by the retention of sweat in contact with the skin.

Inflammation of the skin may be treated with cooling lotions such as Lotion of Witch Hazel or Calamine Lotion with Coal Tar. Compound Calamine Application, Zinc Cream with either Castor Oil or Ichthammol are useful remedies in mild cases. If the rash is pustular, antiseptic dressings of 1:1,000 aqueous solution of aminacrine, 1:500 solution of phenylmercuric nitrate or other mercurial may be applied. If the tissues have been denuded Ichthammol Ointment, Zinc Paste, Compound B.P., Lassar's Paste or Starch Glycerin may be applied spread over lint. If at any stage the irritation from the plaster rash is severe, antipruritics such as benzocaine, menthol or camphor may be incorporated in the remedies used.

Many cases of mild irritation due to adhesive plaster respond to the removal of padding and the application of Compound Benzoin Tincture. Many of these cases are not true plaster dermatitis but merely maceration of the skin by the adhesive plaster mass. Compound Benzoin Tincture does give valuable protection against plaster dermatitis and a sensitive skin may often be protected by applying several coats of the tincture, one coat being allowed to dry before the next is applied. Once a patient has suffered from a plaster dermatitis steps must be taken to modify dressings in such a way as not to provoke further attacks. Non-adhesive dressings or suitable appliances may be devised in many cases or a modification of the forms of padding may give the desired result. Very often plaster dermatitis

124

is a sign that padding is dragging on the skin and a modification in the size or shape of the pad may correct this. To obviate the suction effect of plantar pads in the area posterior to the metatarsal heads, a thin section of felt and adhesive may be removed from the centre of the pad, the piece which has been removed being inverted and replaced so that the adhesive is away from the skin but the thickness of the pad is maintained.

Many dermatological conditions of the skin which are encountered by the chiropodist require immediate reference to a dermatologist. It is important, when choosing a first-aid dressing for patients who are being referred to a skin specialist, to ensure that signs and symptoms which may assist in the diagnosis of the condition should not be masked. For obvious reasons the use of the dyes or any medicament which stains the skin is to be avoided. The dermatologist may also wish to apply bacteriological or mycological tests so that the use of strong antiseptics or strong fungicides immediately prior to consultation with him is contra-indicated. It is suggested that either dry dressings or dressings of saline should be applied or, if an ointment dressing is required, Zinc Paste, Compound B.P.

CHAPTER XVI

THE TREATMENT OF NAIL CONDITIONS

MANY nail conditions call for purely mechanical treatment for the modification of the shape of the nail plate. The same aseptic precautions and antiseptic techniques should be used as for other parts of the foot. Certain nail conditions call for the use of medicaments and those that have not already been considered are discussed below.

To soften a nail plate it should be covered with an emollient ointment on a small piece of lint and then enclosed with waterproof strapping. The nail plate and its surroundings will become soft and macerated after about 7 days. This is a safer and more effective method than the use of salicylic ointments or plasters.

In general it is easier to remove corns and callus from the nail-groove when these are not soft and macerated, so that the use of salicylic acid is contra-indicated. A useful tip before removing corns and callus from a nail groove with the scalpel is to flood the groove with spirit. This shows up the area of callus and any nuclei which may be present are clearly defined. The dressing to be used after the removal of corns and callus from the nail groove depends on the "tone" of the nail sulcus. If it is reasonably dry, Compound Benzoin Tincture may be applied as a routine after-dressing. Iodine oil is also useful, especially if the nail has been packed with felt, cotton wool or amadou. When the nail sulcus is soggy and macerated, a condition which predisposes the formation of corns and callus, an astringent paint may be used. Suitable paints are a 20 per cent solution of silver nitrate in water, Ferric Chloride Solution or 3 per cent salicylic acid in spirit with preference for the latter medicaments. Other astringents, such as formalin, picric acid and chromic acid, may also be used and any general hyperidrotic conditions should be treated. If the sulcus is inflamed as well as being macerated, Witch Hazel Water or half-strength Burow's Solution may be applied.

Collections of debris in the nail groove may be softened with Hydrogen Peroxide Solution. The nail groove may be saturated with the solution and a swab, also saturated, may be placed on it and left in place while other lesions are being treated. The full effect of the action of the Hydrogen Peroxide Solution will not be seen until the operator starts to remove the debris with the excavator. More

Hydrogen Peroxide Solution should be applied after the removal of some of the debris.

Excessive granulation tissue associated with onychocryptosis is best treated with very strong astringents or certain caustics. One of the most commonly used astringents is silver nitrate either as a 50 per cent aqueous solution or as Toughened Silver Nitrate B.P. This should be applied at intervals of 3–4 days. Ferric Chloride Solution, Strong, may also be applied every 3 or 4 days. A crystal of copper sulphate may be used instead of the Toughened Silver Nitrate. When there is much inflammation Witch Hazel Water, or half-strength Burow's Solution, may be applied until the inflammation has subsided, after which a stronger astringent may be used. Malachite green 2 per cent in spirit, very effectively reduces excessive granulation tissue.

Onychia and paronychia should be treated in accordance with the general principles laid down in Chapter X. It must also be borne in mind that a chronic paronychia may be caused by an infection with *Candida albicans*. A preparation of a dye, such as crystal violet, brilliant green or magenta, is useful in these cases, or a solution of phenylmercuric nitrate 1:500 in isopropyl alcohol. The condition should be kept as dry as possible. The treatment of onychomycosis has already been discussed on page 122.

CHAPTER XVII

SURGICAL DRESSINGS

BANDAGES

BANDAGES vary in the material and in the type of weave used in their manufacture.

Cotton and Rubber Elastic Bandage (*Ligamentum Gossypii Elasticum*) B.P.C. consists of a fabric of plain weave in which the warp threads are of singles cotton yarn and combined cotton and rubber yarn and the weft threads are of singles cotton yarn. It stretches lengthwise.

Cotton and Rubber Elastic Net Bandage (*Ligamentum Retis Elasticum*) B.P.C. consists of a net fabric of lace construction in which the warp threads are of combined cotton and rubber yarn and the bobbin threads of mercerized two-fold cotton yarn.

Crêpe Bandage (*Ligamentum Crispi*) B.P.C. is a bandage of plain weave in which the warp yarns are of cotton and wool and the weft yarns of cotton only, giving some lengthwise stretch.

Domette Bandage (*Ligamentum Domettae*) B.P.C. is a union fabric of plain weave, the warp yarns being cotton and the weft yarns being wool. This bandage has a certain amount of transverse stretch.

The above four bandages are used as supporting bandages rather than as a means of applying dressings.

Muslin Bandage (*Ligamentum Sidonis*) B.P.C. is a cotton cloth of plain weave. Muslin bandage is softer and more flexible than open-wove bandage and is especially useful for bandaging toes.

Open-wove Bandage (*Ligamentum Textum Apertum*) B.P.C. is a cotton cloth of plain weave which is used mainly for holding dressings in position. Open-wove bandages are being used less and less in chiropody treatments due to the advent of tubular gauze and elastic bandages, whilst the introduction of the Conforming Bandage has almost replaced the Open-wove Bandage for all the more conventional techniques.

Conforming Bandage, e.g. "Kling" (Johnson & Johnson) is much more loosely woven than the standard Open-wove Bandage and, as the name implies, will more easily conform to the contours of the toes and foot.

128

The disadvantage of the non-stretch type of bandage for the retention of dressings is that it is extremely difficult to produce a satisfactory result which will stay *in situ* over the complex curves encountered when treating the feet. The tubular gauze bandages, e.g. "Tubegauz" (Scholl), "Tubiton" (Seton Products) which are applied by means of a special applicator can more easily be used to produce both an efficient dressing and a neat one. With practice the operator can also produce the exact amount of tension that they require from the tubular bandage by rotating the bandage and applicator whilst applying the material to the foot. There is now a complete range of sizes to suit any part or size of foot encountered to produce the most efficient result. It is also conveniently used by the patient when required to replace dressings.

Along the same lines there has, within the last few years, been available *Tubular Elastic Bandage*—"Tubigrip" (Seton Products)—which is produced in several sizes, some of which have applications in chiropody treatments. It can usefully be employed to retain dressings or support where required, and also be used as a means of producing anchorage to the foot for removable pads, etc. There is also now available this same elasticated bandage which includes polyurethane foam for about half the circumference of the bandage. It can very quickly be cut in lengths to produce protective covers or simple pads, or even carriers for the addition of other padding materials.

Along very similar lines, using the above described tubular bandage as a base on which to form polyurethane foam, there are available "tubes" of foam formed on to the bandage of sizes appropriate to the range of normal toe sizes. These can very quickly be cut to a length convenient to the toe concerned, and form a quick method of producing a simple pad. The polyurethane foam is a good thermal insulator and is therefore suggested when protection from excessive friction is required. It also has applications in the treatment of chilblains, etc.

Plaster of Paris Bandage (*Ligamentum Calcii Sulphatis*) B.P.C. consists of bleached cotton cloth impregnated with Exsiccated Calcium Sulphate treated with suitable adhesives in order to attach it to the fabric. It is used for the taking of negative casts in the preparation of various appliances.

Rayon and Rubber Elastic Bandage (*Ligamentum Rayon Elasticum*) B.P.C. consists of a fabric in which the warp threads are of two-fold rayon staple fibre and combined cotton and rubber yarn, and the weft threads are of rayon yarn only. It may be used instead of Cotton Elastic Bandage.

Zinc Oxide Elastic Self-adhesive Bandage (*Ligamentum Elasticum Adhesivum*) B.P.C. consists of elastic cloth spread evenly with a self-adhesive plaster mass containing at least 20 per cent of zinc oxide.

In *Half-spread Zinc Oxide Elastic Self-adhesive Bandage* B.P.C. and *Ventilated Zinc Oxide Self-adhesive Bandage* B.P.C. portions of the elastic cloth, not exceeding 50 per cent of the whole, are left unspread.

COTTON WOOL

Absorbent Cotton Wool (*Gossypium Absorbens*) B.P.C. consists of bleached, carded cotton fibres, loosened and separated to form a mass of soft white filaments. It readily absorbs water but loses much of its absorbency if it is medicated. Cotton wool has many and varied uses in the practice of chiropody which do not require discussion here.

Capsicum Cotton Wool (*Gossypium Capsici*) B.P.C. is cotton wool impregnated with the oleoresin of capsicum and with methyl salicylate. It is tinted orange-brown. It is a useful rubefacient combining direct rubefacient action with heat-insulating properties.

Sterile cotton wool is now fairly readily available, generally in the form of cotton wool balls. Probably the most useful pack from the chiropodist's point of view is the pack of two in sealed envelopes. Sterile cotton wool is required for the special occasion rather than for general use.

GAUZE

Absorbent Gauze (*Carbasus Absorbens*) B.P.C. consists of cotton cloth of a plain weave, having an average of not less than 19 threads an inch to the warp and not less than 15 threads an inch to the weft. Gauze may be medicated but it loses much of its absorbency when it is so treated. Absorbent gauze may be used as a dry dressing to absorb discharges from wounds, or as a medium for the application of medicaments in liquid and semi-liquid form. Gauze may be obtained in ribbon from *Absorbent Ribbon Gauze* (*Carbasus Absorbens in Taenia*) B.P.C. in various widths. Ribbon gauze is normally supplied in bottles with a small screw cap set in the lid.

The official medicated gauzes are:

Paraffin Gauze Dressing (*Curatio Carbasi Paraffini*) B.P.C. syn.

Tulle Gras Dressing, consists of bleached cotton cloth which is packed into metal containers, impregnated with yellow soft paraffin to which 1·25 per cent of Peru Balsam has been added, and the whole sterilized by heating to 135° C. for thirty minutes. The pieces of gauze are available in several sizes. Tulle gras is also used in chiropody as an emollient, squares of the material being held in place over an affected area, often with an elastic self-adhesive bandage.

Proprietary preparations similar to the above are "Jelonet" (Smith & Nephew), "Nonad Tulle" (Allen & Hanburys) and "Petronet" (Dalmas).

Gauze and Capsicum Cotton Tissue (Tela Carbasi et Gossypii Capsici) B.P.C. consists of a thick layer of capsicum cotton wool enclosed in tubular absorbent gauze, tinted orange-brown with a suitable dye. It is rubefacient and heat-insulating.

Probably the most important developments in this field have been the recent production and availability of individual prepackaged sterile gauze swabs and of other non-adherent dressings. One of the problems with conventional Absorbent Gauze, whether sterilized or not, was that it often adhered to any discharge from minor cuts and ulcers encountered on the feet. There are now available several non-adherent dressings which are individually packaged, sterile and a size convenient to the chiropodist. The product is a highly absorbent acrylic and cotton fibre pad, bonded to a very thin polyester film which is perforated. It should be placed with the plastic film to the wound and can readily be lifted off without sticking or disturbing the healing processes. Conventional dressings can be used in the usual manner. "Melolin Xa" (Smith & Nephew) is individually packed and the sizes most useful to the chiropodist are 5 cm. × 5 cm. (2 in. × 2 in.) and 10 cm. × 10 cm. (4 in. × 4 in.).

LINT

Absorbent Lint (Linteum Absorbens) B.P.C. is a cotton cloth of plain weave. On one side of the cloth the warp yarns are raised to form a nap. Lint may be used for the application of wet dressings or of ointments and pastes, the medicament being spread on the plain side of the lint. Lint may also be used as a dry dressing, with the plain side against the wound.

Euflavine Lint (Linteum Euflavine) B.P.C. contains from 0·0075 to 0·2 per cent of Euflavine.

PLASTERS

Self-adhesive or pressure-sensitive plasters are manufactured by spreading the pressure-sensitive mass on to various materials. The mass consists of a cohesive agent such as para rubber, crêpe rubber, smoked sheet rubber or a synthetic rubber of high quality, with a tackifier, which is a natural or synthetic resin such as colophony, a plasticizer and a filler which must not be more than 25 per cent of the whole. Zinc oxide 20–30 per cent is incorporated in most self-adhesive plasters. The pressure-sensitive mass may be spread on a variety of materials, for instance on plain holland to provide the ordinary chiropodist's strapping, or on cloths woven in such a way that the roll has either a lengthwise or transverse stretch. The self-adhesive plaster mass may also be spread on plastic film, stockinette, wool felt, sponge rubber, fleecy web, etc., all of which have their particular uses in chiropody[1].

Capsicum and belladonna may be incorporated in the plaster mass to make a rubefacient plaster and salicylic acid to make a keratolytic one.

Extension Plaster B.P.C. syn. Extension Strapping, consists of elastic cloth which stretches in the direction of the weft, spread evenly with self-adhesive plaster mass containing zinc oxide.

Perforated Plastic Self-adhesive Plaster B.P.C. consists of an extensible perforated plastic film, permeable to air and water vapour, spread evenly with a self-adhesive plaster mass.

Waterproof Plastic Self-adhesive Plaster B.P.C. consists of an extensible water-impermeable plastic film spread with a self-adhesive plaster mass.

Waterproof Micro-porous Plastic Self-adhesive Plaster B.P.C. consists of an extensible water-impermeable plastic film, permeable to water vapour and air, spread with a self-adhesive plaster mass.

Salicylic Acid Self-adhesive Plaster B.P.C.—see Salicylic Acid.

Zinc Oxide Elastic Self-adhesive Plaster B.P.C. consists of elastic cloth which stretches in the direction of the warp, spread with self-adhesive plaster mass containing zinc oxide.

Zinc Oxide Self-adhesive Plaster B.P.C. consists of a suitable cloth spread evenly with a self-adhesive plaster mass containing zinc oxide.

---

[1] Some modern adhesive plasters use other adhesive materials which are less likely to cause skin-reactions.

WOOL

Animal Wool for Chiropody B.P.C. is wool obtained from the back of the sheep, *Ovis aries*. Foreign substances and animal grease are removed by scouring, washing and combing. The quality of the wool is 46's to 56's, Bradford classification, with an average length of not less than 5 inches, the longest fibres being not less than 9 inches long.

Wool is very hygroscopic, absorbing up to 50 per cent of moisture, but it has a normal moisture regain of $18\frac{1}{4}$ per cent. Animal Wool, wrapped loosely round the toes, serves to redistribute pressure away from a painful corn. It must be remembered that, being wool, it will shrink considerably when moist. Because it shrinks, and also because it is not sterile, it should not be used to secure wet dressings in place.

AMADOU

This material is prepared from a fungus *Boletus igniarius* of the order *Basidiomycetes*, which grows on old trees, especially birch and beech. The fungus is cut into slices and steeped in a solution of nitre. The preparation of amadou was carried out chiefly in the Black Forest region of Germany, although the fungus is found also in Scotland and in other European countries. Amadou is a tough, strong substance which remains soft under moist conditions. It is used for packing nail grooves and has the advantage that the nitre content gives it an astringent action. The original use of Amadou was as a tinder.

PLASTIC FILM DRESSINGS

These are a synthetic organic compound of acrylic resin dissolved in ethyl acetate and a plasticizer, developed for direct application on to the skin. The two most readily available, in aerosol dispensers are "Nobecutane" (Duncan, Flockhart & Evans), and "Octaflex" (Ward, Blenkinsop) which has the added advantage of antiseptic properties.

They have the following properties:

(a) impervious to bacteria;

(b) transparent—allows inspection of painted area;

(c) high tensile strength—sufficiently elastic to allow normal joint movements;

(d) waterproof, but permeable to air and water, do not impede healthy granulation;

(*e*) not readily affected by soap and water;

(*f*) easily removed by the use of a solvent;

(*g*) non-irritant.

In chiropody practice they can be utilized in many ways, some of which include:

(*a*) as a thick film adhering to the skin to reduce friction;

(*b*) in conjunction with gauze dressings as a method of retention;

(*c*) as false toe nails in conjunction with gauze;

(*d*) as a post-operative application to minimize reaction to plaster spread on felts and strappings.

MISCELLANEOUS

Chiropodists also employ as dressings a wide variety of materials from very soft sponge rubber, latex or plastic foams to hard-compressed felt in order to redirect and redistribute pressure on the feet. These materials are constantly being improved and new materials introduced and these types of dressings have not yet been standardized in the technical sense. They are selected for their mechanical attributes and a description of them lies outside the scope of this work.

PART TWO

MONOGRAPHS

INCOMPATIBILITY

Incompatibility may be:

1. Chemical, i.e. two drugs cannot be administered together without their forming a new chemical compound. In some cases drugs which are incompatible are deliberately administered together, for example nitric acid and phenol in the treatment of warts. In other cases the application of an incompatible substance which will form some harmless new compound is used to inhibit the action of a drug, for instance sodium chloride is used to stop the action of silver nitrate. Sometimes, however, when two drugs are administered together they form a poisonous, or otherwise dangerous new compound, or merely make a mess, as when salicylic acid or the salicylates come into contact with ferric´ chloride, or Compound Benzoin Tincture comes into contact with water.

2. Physical, i.e. the physical nature of the drugs prevents them from being applied together, e.g. an oily solution with a watery solution.

3. Physiological, i.e. two drugs may exert a directly opposite pharmacological action to one another and thus cancel out their effects.

The more important incompatibilities of each drug are listed in the following monographs.

The abbreviation R.P. is used to denote "return period".

ACETIC ACID

Glacial Acetic Acid (*Acidum Aceticum Glaciale*) B.P. contains not less than 99 per cent of $CH_3 \cdot COOH$. Glacial acetic acid is a colourless liquid with a distinctive vinegary odour. Below 14·3° C. it crystallizes to form colourless crystals, so that on a very cold day it may be necessary, before use, to warm the bottle in the hands. On no account should water be added in order to dissolve the crystals.

Glacial acetic acid is a weak acid which is mildly caustic in its action. It may be used as a paint in the treatment of hard or vascular corns, or of verruca pedis (R.P. 14–21 days). A method of treatment in the case of verruca pedis is first, to saturate the growth with glacial acetic acid, which should be rubbed well in, and then, to rub the lesion with a stick of Toughened Silver Nitrate B.P. which has been moistened with water. Two or three further applications of glacial acetic acid are made alternately with the silver nitrate stick to com-

137

plete a single treatment. (Minimum R.P. is 4 days.) This is a very mild method of treatment.

Glacial Acetic Acid may also be used as a neutralizing agent following treatment of a wart with Potassium hydroxide.

Acetic Acid (*Acidum Aceticum*) B.P. contains approximately 33 per cent of CH_3COOH w/w and must therefore be carefully distinguished from Glacial Acetic Acid when ordering. It is not widely used in chiropody but has been employed as a fungicide in the treatment of onychomycosis.

Other Acids

Malic Acid, Hydroxysuccinic Acid, $C_4H_6O_5$ is used in the proprietary "Aserbine" (Horlicks) which is available as a Cream containing Malic Acid 250 mg., the Malic Acid Ester of Propylene Glycol 160 mg., Benzoic Acid 25 mg., and Salicylic Acid 5 mg. in each 100 grammes: or as a solution containing 1·53 per cent of Malic Acid, 1·05 per cent of the Malic Acid Ester of Propylene Glycol, 0·15 per cent of Benzoic Acid and 0·03 per cent of Salicylic Acid in Propylene Glycol and Rose Water.

"Aserbine" is used for the treatment of indolent ulcers with heavy sloughing. The area is first swabbed with "Aserbine" solution followed by an application of the cream on non-adherent gauze. "Aserbine" should not be brought into contact with metallic surfaces.

Tartaric Acid B.P. ($C_4H_6O_6$) is used in the preparation of effervescent foot-baths.

ACETONE

Acetone (*Acetonum*) B.P.C. is dimethyl ketone $CH_3CO \cdot CH_3$, a colourless, light, inflammable liquid with a distinctive odour less pungent than that of ether. It should be stored in dark, glass-stoppered bottles which prevent access of moisture. It has a flash point[1] of $-17°$ C.

Acetone is a solvent and is used on cotton wool swabs for cleansing the skin prior to operating. Its efficiency as a cleanser depends on the vigour with which the swabbing is done. Acetone readily dissolves fats and resins and is used as a solvent for pyroxylin in the preparation of Collodions (see Pyroxylin).

Acetone is said to have a slight hardening effect on the skin, for which purpose, however, it is not used. Its hardening action does not affect its use as a solvent. Acetone varies in its efficiency as a solvent

---

[1] Flash point is the temperature at which the vapour from a volatile substance becomes inflammable.

of various brands of adhesive plasters. For the removal of fresh plaster marks from the skin acetone is more useful than ether because it is less volatile and the adhesive, therefore, remains in solution. On the other hand, if ether is used, the solvent evaporates so rapidly that some adhesive is left on the skin. Acetone is safer to use than ether and its odour is often found to be less offensive to the patient.

ACRIFLAVINE (see Amino-acridines)

ADRENALINE

Adrenaline (*Adrenalina*) B.P. syn. Epinephrine
$$(C_6H_3(OH)_2 \cdot CHOH \cdot CH_2 \cdot NH \cdot CH_3)$$
is the active principle of the medulla of the suprarenal gland.

Adrenaline, which may be prepared synthetically, occurs as a white crystalline powder sparingly soluble in water, insoluble in alcohol or ether.

Adrenaline Solution (*Liquor Adrenalinae*) B.P. contains Adrenaline Acid Tartrate 0·18 per cent (equivalent to Adrenaline 1:1,000) with Chlorbutol, Sodium Metabisulphide and Sodium Chloride in water.

Externally, adrenaline is used as Adrenaline Solution B.P. as a haemostatic and vasoconstrictor. It has a direct action on the blood vessels. A haemorrhage which has been arrested with adrenaline may be dressed with any of the usual wound prophylactics.

On no account should adrenaline or any other vasoconstrictor be used in conjunction with a local anaesthetic injection because in a digit there is a danger of ischaemia which may lead to gangrene.

"Lloyd's Adrenaline Cream" (Howard Lloyd) is a stabilized buffered cream containing 0·02 per cent adrenaline. This may be applied to areas of callus following the removal of thickened stratum corneum.

THE ALCOHOLS

In organic chemistry the term *Alcohol* is used to describe a number of compounds. The technical definition of an alcohol is a substance having one or more —OH (hydroxyl) groups attached to a saturated carbon atom. (A saturated carbon atom is one with all its valencies satisfied.) The carbon atom or atoms must not form part of a carboxyl group:

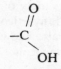

The alcohols are classified according to the number of hydroxyl groups they contain:

Class	Formula	Name
Monohydric	C_2H_5OH	Ethyl alcohol
Dihydric	CH_2OH | CH_2OH	Ethylene glycol
Trihydric	CH_2OH | $CHOH$ | CH_2OH	Glycerin or glycerol

Thus the definition *Alcohol* in organic chemistry covers a very wide range of compounds.

Here the concern is with a group of monohydric alcohols having the general formula $C_nN_{2n+1}OH$. They include:

Name	Formula
Methyl alcohol or methanol	CH_3OH
Ethyl alcohol or ethanol	$CH_3 \cdot CH_2 \cdot OH$
Propyl alcohol or propanol	$CH_3 \cdot (CH_2)_2 \cdot OH$
Isopropyl alcohol or isopropanol	$(CH_3)_2 \cdot CH \cdot OH$
Cetyl alcohol	$CH_3 \cdot (CH_2)_{14} \cdot CH_2 \cdot OH$
Stearyl alcohol	$CH_3 \cdot (CH_2)_{16} \cdot CH_2 \cdot OH$

It will be noticed that propyl alcohol and isopropyl alcohol both correspond to the general formula C_3H_7OH. The arrangement of the atoms within the molecule is slightly different in the two substances:

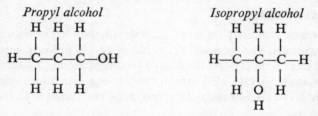

The term *alcohol* may have a variety of meanings according to the context in which it is used. Ethyl alcohol C_2H_5OH is frequently called simply "alcohol" and is also known as "spirit". If a substance is described as being "soluble in alcohol", it means that it is soluble in ethyl alcohol.

Ethyl Alcohol

Alcohol (95 per cent) B.P. consists of a mixture of ethyl alcohol, C_2H_5OH and water. It is a transparent, colourless liquid with a characteristic odour and a burning taste. It contains 94·7–95·2 per cent v/v or 92·0–92·7 per cent w/w of C_2H_5OH.

When alcohol is mixed with water, there is a contraction in volume and a rise in temperature.

Alcohol (90 per cent) (*Spiritus Rectificatus*), consists of 947 ml. of Alcohol (95 per cent) diluted to 1,000 ml. with water.

Proof Spirit (*Spiritus Tenuior*) is defined as that which at 51° F. weighs exactly 12/13ths as much as an equal volume of distilled water. It contains 57·1 per cent v/v of C_2H_5OH. Spirits are described as being so many degrees over or under proof spirit according to the quantity of distilled water which must be added to, or deducted from, 100 volumes of the sample in order to produce proof spirit. Thus 100 volumes of 90 per cent alcohol contain as much C_2H_5OH as 158 volumes of proof spirit, so that to bring 100 volumes of 90 per cent alcohol to the same strength as proof spirit 58 volumes of water would have to be added, therefore 90 per cent alcohol is said to be 58° over proof, or 58 O.P.

Dehydrated Alcohol (*Alcohol Dehydratum*) B.P. contains not less than 99·4 per cent v/v of C_2H_5OH. Owing to its great affinity for water it is a powerful dehydrating agent. It is expensive to prepare, deteriorates quickly, and has little to recommend its use in chiropody.

Industrial Methylated Spirit (*Spiritus Methylatus Industrialis*) B.P. syn. I.M.S. is a mixture, prepared by a legally authorized methylator, of 19 volumes of Alcohol (95 per cent) with 1 volume of approved wood naphtha (see Methyl Alcohol). It is known as 66 O.P. Industrial Methylated Spirit. It is a colourless, transparent, mobile and volatile liquid with a burning taste.

Other strengths of Industrial Methylated Spirit are available, e.g. Absolute Industrial Methylated Spirit which is 74 O.P. and which contains less than 1 per cent of water, and also 64 O.P. Industrial Methylated Spirit.

Industrial Methylated Spirit (*Acetone Free*) (*Spiritus Methylatus Industrialis Sine Acetono*) B.P.C. is the same as the above but is free from acetone. It is used to prepare solutions of iodine for external use: iodine forms an irritant compound with acetone.

Industrial Methylated Spirit B.P. is used to prepare surgical spirit:

Surgical Spirit (*Spiritus Chirugicalis*) B.P.C.: Castor Oil 2·5 per cent, Methyl Salicylate 0·5 per cent, Ethyl Phthalate 2 per cent, Industrial Methylated Spirit to 100 per cent.

The use of Industrial Methylated Spirit in preparing the above formula has been approved by the Board of Customs and Excise.

The following formula has also been approved by the Board:

Foot Spirit (Spiritus Pedibus): Salicylic Acid 3 per cent, Methyl Salicylate 0·5 per cent, Diethyl Phthalate 1 per cent, Industrial Methylated Spirit to 100 per cent.

The Uses of Alcohol. Alcohol is antiseptic, astringent, dehydrating and is a solvent. As a pre-operative cleansing agent the action of alcohol depends rather on its power as a solvent than on its antiseptic qualities. The efficiency of its action is controlled by the vigour with which the swabbing is carried out. Industrial Methylated Spirit may be used for pre-operative cleansing and may be employed also, on a cotton wool swab, for wiping knives and other instruments immediately before and after use. When the skin is wet with spirit, corns, callus and similar lesions show a clearly defined line of demarcation between these and healthy skin. Alcohol is at its maximum antiseptic strength at a concentration of 70 per cent: its antiseptic efficiency decreases at greater and lesser concentrations. Antiseptics dissolved in I.M.S. may be used when a drying and slightly astringent action is required on moist or soggy wounds. 70 per cent strength Isopropyl alcohol is increasingly being used as a solvent in lieu of I.M.S. I.M.S., itself an astringent, may be used as a solvent for various astringent medicaments for external use. The most common example is 3 per cent Salicylic Acid in spirit employed as in the formula quoted above.

Evaporating Lotion B.P.C. 1954 contains 12·5 per cent of Alcohol (90 per cent) or I.M.S., Ammonium Chloride 3·43 per cent in water to 100 per cent. It is a cooling lotion depending on evaporation to produce coldness.

Methyl Alcohol (*Alcohol Methylicum*) syn. Methanol is a colourless liquid with an alcoholic odour and a burning taste. It is a poison, causing blindness if taken internally. Methyl alcohol is used to denature alcohol, to render it unfit for drinking and therefore free from duty. Wood naphtha, which is used to prepare I.M.S., contains 60·9 per cent of methyl alcohol, CH_3OH.

Isopropyl Alcohol (*Alcohol Isopropylicum*) B.P. Trade name: "Avantine" (Howard, Ilford) is a clear, colourless liquid with a spirituous odour and a burning taste.

Isopropyl alcohol may be used as a pre-operative cleanser at 30 per cent strength and in the preparation of lotions for external application. It is being increasingly used as a solvent for local antiseptics such as the acridines and phenylmercuric nitrate. Wherever possible it should be used in lieu of Industrial Methylated Spirit.

Cetyl Alcohol, Stearyl Alcohol

Cetostearyl Alcohol (Alcohol Cetostearylicum) B.P. is a mixture of solid aliphatic alcohols, chiefly cetyl alcohol $CH_3 \cdot (CH_2)_{14} \cdot CH_2OH$ and stearyl alcohol $CH_3 \cdot (CH_2)_{16} \cdot CH_2OH$. It is a white or cream-coloured mass insoluble in water but soluble in ether and alcohol.

Cetostearyl alcohol is of little value as an emulsifying agent when used alone but, in conjunction with a hydrophilic substance, such as a sulphated fatty alcohol, it produces stable oil-in-water emulsions.

Cetostearyl alcohol is an ingredient of Emulsifying Wax, Paraffin Ointment and Simple Ointment.

Emulsifying Wax (Cera Emulsificans) B.P. consists of 90 grammes of Cetostearyl Alcohol, 10 grammes of Sodium Lauryl Sulphate with 4 ml. of water.

Emulsifying wax mixes readily with hot water to form a Cream and also forms oil-in-water emulsions with fatty or paraffin bases. This type of emulsion is often used as a protective barrier-cream. Oil-in-water creams are suitable vehicles for water-soluble medicaments and also have a cooling effect due to evaporation of the continuous watery phase from the skin. They assist the penetration of the dissolved medicament and, in general, a lower percentage of the drug is required in an oil-in-water emulsion than in a fatty ointment base.

Emulsifying Ointment (Unguentum Emulsificans) B.P. consists of 30 per cent of Emulsifying Wax, 50 per cent of White Soft Paraffin and 20 per cent of Liquid Paraffin.

Aqueous Cream (Unguentum Emulsificans Aquosum) Simple Cream B.P. consists of 30 per cent of Emulsifying Ointment, 0·1 per cent of Chlorocresol with Distilled Water to 100 per cent.

Paraffin Ointment (Unguentum Paraffini) B.P. consists of 2 per cent of Beeswax, 3 per cent of Hard Paraffin, 5 per cent of Cetostearyl Alcohol and 90 per cent of White or Yellow Soft Paraffin.

Simple Ointment (Unguentum Simplex) B.P. consists of 5 per cent of Wool Fat, 5 per cent of Hard Paraffin, 5 per cent of Cetostearyl Alcohol and 85 per cent of White or Yellow Soft Paraffin.

Paraffin Ointment and Simple Ointment are frequently used as ointment bases and are themselves useful emollients.

Cetyl alcohol is an ingredient of another valuable emollient cream, viz.: 4 per cent of Cetyl Alcohol, 6 per cent of Glycerin and 90 per cent of White Soft Paraffin. This cream 'is especially useful for the hands following the defatting of the skin with detergents such as cetrimide. It renders the skin smooth and velvety rather than slippery.

"Lanette Wax SX" (Ronsheim & Moore) is an anionic self-emulsifying wax consisting of a partially sulphated mixture of cetyl and stearyl alcohols used to prepare oil-in-water emulsions. It is said to assist absorption of medicaments incorporated in the emulsion.

ALUM

Alum (*Alumen*) B.P. may be either Potash Alum, potassium aluminium sulphate $KAl(SO_4)_2 \cdot 12H_2O$, or Ammonia Alum, ammonium aluminium sulphate $NH_4Al(SO_4)_2 \cdot 12H_2O$. They occur as colourless crystals or as a white powder. They are soluble 1 part in 7 parts of water, 1 in 3 of glycerin, but are insoluble in alcohol.

Alum is incompatible with the salts of mercury and with borax.

Alum is used as an astringent and haemostatic. It coagulates protein and has a hardening action on the skin. A saturated solution in water may be employed in cases of hyperidrosis or bromidrosis either as a paint or as a foot-bath (3 teaspoonfuls to the pint). Alum powder may be used on soft corns, on relaxed nail sulci and on hypergranulation tissue, when it acts as a powerful astringent.

Burnt Alum is prepared by heating potash alum until it has lost 45–46 per cent of its weight.

Burnt Alum is sometimes used on hypergranulation tissue but it is very painful if any of the powder finds its way into a breach in the skin.

ALUMINIUM ACETATE

Aluminium Acetate Solution (*Liquor Aluminii Acetatis*) B.P.C. syn. Burow's solution is a saturated solution of basic aluminium acetate containing the equivalent of about 13 per cent of aluminium acetate. It is prepared by dissolving aluminium sulphate (225 grammes) in water (600 ml.) and adding acetic acid (250 ml.). To this mixture is added calcium carbonate (100 grammes) in water (150 ml.). The final product is allowed to stand in a cool place for 24 hours and is then filtered.

Burow's solution is used as an antiseptic and astringent lotion, generally diluted one part to three parts of water. It is generally used in chiropody for the reduction of inflammation but it is also suitable for use on suppurating wounds. The diluted solution may be applied as an evaporating compress in cases of acute bursitis, either infective or traumatic (R.P. 1–2 days). The 1:3 dilution may also be applied daily as a dressing in the hyperaemic stage of chilblains or as an antiseptic and astringent lotion in cases of plaster dermatitis. Diluted with an equal volume of water, Burow's solution may be employed as a paint in cases of the inflamed type of hyperidrosis and bromidrosis.

"Domeboro Tablets" (Dome) contain aluminium sulphate and calcium acetate; dissolved in water they produce a modified Burow's solution containing calcium sulphate in fine suspension.

ANALGESICS, LOCAL

The first local analgesic to be introduced into clinical practice was cocaine in 1884. Its analgesic properties were discovered by accident by Freud and Koller while attempting to cure a friend of morphine addiction. Cocaine is an alkaloid derived from Erythroxylum coca. Most local analgesics in current use are derivatives of cocaine. Many have an ester structure similar to that of cocaine; some have an amide linkage. Most have the suffix "-caine" in their name.

The typical local analgesic structure is represented by procaine

$$H_2N - \text{(benzene ring)} - CO - O - CH_2 - CH_2 - N \underset{C_2H_5}{\overset{C_2H_5}{<}}$$

| Lipophilic group | Intermediate chain | Hydrophilic group |

Both the potency and toxicity of a local analgesic are largely determined by the length of the intermediate chain which is usually either an ester or an amide linkage. A longer chain may be more potent but may also be more toxic. Structural re-arrangement of the groupings is responsible for more effective analgesic action. The following are criteria for clinically acceptable analgesics: complete reversibility of of action; absence of local tissue toxicity; high potency; short time for onset of anaesthesia; sufficient duration of action; stability during sterilization process and on storage. In principle the lowest concentration and least quantity which will give adequate anaesthesia should be used.

Amethocaine Hydrochloride is an analgesic of the ester type which, in chiropody, is only used topically.

Amethocaine Hydrochloride (*Amethocainae Hydrochloridum*) B.P. syn. Tetracaine Hydrochloride: [$C_4H_9NH \cdot C_6H_4 \cdot CO \cdot O \cdot CH_2 \cdot CH_2 \cdot N(CH_3)_2$] HCl is a white crystalline powder soluble 1 part in 8 of water and 1 part in 40 of alcohol.

Amethocaine is a local anaesthetic which has a considerable surface action when applied externally especially to mucous membranes. Generally a 1 per cent solution is applied on a cotton wool swab which is left in position for about five minutes before operating begins. It is very effective when it reaches the nerve endings but it is difficult to obtain sufficient penetration. It is useful on broken surfaces and will, for instance, take away the pain of a haemostatic applied to a wound. It has proved disappointing in nail groove work chiefly owing to the difficulty of obtaining sufficient penetration. "Anethaine Ointment" (Glaxo) contains Amethocaine Hydrochloride 1 per cent in a water-miscible base.

"Locan Ointment' (Duncan, Flockhart & Evans) contains Amethocaine 0·8 per cent, Amylocaine 1·0 per cent and Cinchocaine 0·4 per cent in a vanishing cream base. "Polycrest Antiseptic Cream" (Nicholas Laboratories) contains Benzocaine 5 per cent, Phenylmercuric nitrate 0·25 per cent and Amethocaine Hydrochloride 0·5 per cent in a non-greasy base.

Benzocaine is another local analgesic of the ester type. It is used topically as a surface anaesthetic, see Benzocaine page 151.

The four local analgesics authorised for Chiropodists who have been appropriately trained to use by injection are all of the amide type. They are less readily metabolised then the ester type but are slightly more liable to produce untoward effects. All are used in plain solution, i.e. without adrenaline. They are:

Bupivacaine Hydrochloride B.P. Prop: Marcain. [$CH_3 \cdot (CH_2)_3 \cdot C_5H_9N \cdot CO \cdot NH \cdot C_6H_3 \cdot (CH_3)_2)$] HCl, H_2O is a white odourless crystalline powder, soluble 1 in 25 of water and 1 in 8 of alcohol.

Bupivacaine is a long-acting local analgesic, similar to lignocaine and mepivacaine but it is from 2 to 4 times more potent and may therefore be used in lower strengths. Its onset time is similar to that of Lignocaine, but its duration of action is longer. The maximum dose is 2 mg. per Kg. body weight per 24 hours.

Lignocaine Hydrochloride B.P. Prop: Lidothesin, Lignostab,

Xylocaine, Xylotox, [(CH$_3$)$_2$·C$_6$H$_3$·NH·CO·CH$_2$·N·(C$_2$H$_5$)$_2$] HCl, H$_2$O is a white crystalline powder which is highly soluble in both water and alcohol.

Lignocaine may be used either by injection or as a topical application. Introduced in 1948 it is now one of the most widely used of local analgesics. In equal concentrations it is more effective than the ester type analgesic Procaine being more rapid in onset and longer in duration. It has a low allergenicity. Below 0·5 per cent its toxicity is similar to that of Prilocaine but in higher strengths it is more toxic. Local irritant effects are rare. Solutions exceeding 2 per cent concentrations are rarely used and the maximum safe dosage is 200 mg. per 24 hours. Any toxic effects occur rapidly in 2–3 minutes after injection and are generally due to overdosage. Symptoms include drowsiness, brachycardia, muscular twitching, hypotension and respiratory arrest. Allergic reactions and anaphylactic shock have been reported following incorrect dosage or accidental intravenous injection. Lignocaine has a slight vaso-dilatatory effect. For topical use lignocaine is used as a 2 per cent gel or 5 per cent cream.

Prilocaine Hydrochloride B.P. Prop: Citanest [CH$_3$·C$_6$H$_5$·NH·CO·CH(CH$_3$)·NH· (CH$_2$)$_2$·CH$_3$] HCl occurs as white crystals or white crystalline powder which is soluble 1 in 5 of water and 1 in 6 of alchol.

Prilocaine is a local analgesic with similar properties to Lignocaine but it is about 50 per cent less toxic. It should be used with caution in patients with anaemia, cardiac failure or impaired respiratory function. It causes less vaso-dilatation than Lignocaine and has about 25 per cent longer lasting effect. The maximum dosage is 200 mg. per 24 hours. Overdosage may give rise to methaemoglobinaemia. It should not be used on pregnant women.

Mepivacaine Hydrochloride U.S.N.F. Prop: Carbocaine [CH$_3$·C$_5$H$_9$N·CO·NH·C$_6$H$_3$ (CH$_3$)$_2$] HCl is a white odourless powder which is very soluble in water and soluble 1 in 10 of alcohol. It is incompatible with alkalies. Again Mepivacaine has properties similar to those of Lignocaine. It is more rapid in onset and lasts approximately 20 per cent longer. Tissue toxicity is low up to 4 per cent strength. The maximum dosage is 400 mg. per 24 hours. It has the advantage of not having any vaso-dilatory properties. Any adverse reactions occur 8–10 minutes after injection. Mepivacaine is the most recently introduced of the local analgesics and to date no specific contra indication to its use are listed.

The maximum doses quoted above are in all four cases, absolute maxima. The maximum dose required in clinical chiropody is well below those figures generally by the order of five.

AMINO-ACRIDINES

Although there are numerous references to the amino-acridines, particularly aminacrine and proflavine throughout this reprint, these drugs are no longer available and the monograph on local analgesics has been substituted in the text.

AMMONIUM BICARBONATE

Aromatic Spirit of Ammonia (*Liquor Ammoniae Aromaticus*) B.P. syn. Spirit of Sal Volatile consists of Ammonium Bicarbonate (25 grammes) dissolved in a mixture of Strong Solution of Ammonia (60 ml.), Lemon Oil (5 ml.), Nutmeg Oil (3 ml.), 90 per cent Alcohol (750 ml.) and Distilled Water to produce 1,000 ml.

Sal Volatile is used internally for faintness: 3 ml. (half a teaspoonful) to a medicine glass, 50 ml. (2 oz.), of water. It may also be applied externally to insect bites. Since it contains ammonia, Sal Volatile will remove fresh stains of the coal tar dyes, such as crystal violet, fuchsin, etc., from the skin.

Smelling salts containing ammonium bicarbonate help in warding off faintness.

ANTIBIOTICS USED TOPICALLY

Antibiotics are controlled by the Therapeutic Substances Act and are available only on prescription signed by a Registered Medical Practitioner.

Bacitracin B.P. is a wide-spectrum antibiotic, active against many Gram-positive and a few Gram-negative bacteria. It is used mainly as an external application.

Neomycin Sulphate B.P. is a wide-spectrum antibiotic, active against a very wide range of organisms. It is inactive against fungi and viruses. Neomycin consists of two isomers, neomycin B and neomycin C. About 10–15 per cent of neomycin C is present in commercial Neomycin. *Framycetin* consists of neomycin B with a small proportion of neomycin C.

Neomycin Cream B.P.C. contains 0·5 per cent of Neomycin Sulphate. The cream is prepared with Cetomacrogol Emulsifying Ointment as Neomycin is incompatible with the anionic emulgents in Aqueous Cream:

"Cicatrin" (Calmic) Cream and Powder contain Neomycin Sulphate, Bacitracin Zinc, with amino-acids. For promoting healing in wounds and ulcers.

"Dermamed" (Medo Chemicals) is an ointment containing Neomycin and Bacitracin.

"Graneodin" (Squibb) is an ointment containing Neomycin and Gramicidin.

"Myciguent" (Upjohn) is an ointment containing Neomycin.

"My-San" (Nu-San Ltd.) is a sterile non-adherent dressing of acetate cloth impregnated with Neomycin and Bithionol.

"Negamycin Dusting-powder with Amino-acids" (Therapharm) contains Neomycin, Gramicidin with Amino-acids.

"Neobacrin Tulle" (Glaxo) is a tulle dressing impregnated with Neomycin and Bacitracin Zinc.

"Neolate Polyantibiotic Powder" (Therapharm) contains Neomycin Sulphate and Bacitracin Zinc. Also available with amino-acids.

"Neomycin Dusting Powder" (Therapharm) contains 0·5 per cent Neomycin.

"Nivebaxin" (Boots) is a dusting-powder containing Neomycin Bacitracin Zinc and Polymixin.

"Rikospray Antibiotic" (Riker) is an aerosol spray containing Neomycin, Bacitracin Zinc and Colistin Sulphate.

"Trimycin Dusting Powder" (Therapharm) contains Neomycin, Bacitracin Zinc and Polymixin B.

"Cortibiotic Skin Ointment" (Roussel) contains Framycetin, Gramicidin and Prednisolone.

"Framygen" (Fisons) is a Framycetin Cream (0·5 per cent)

"Framycort" is available as an ointment containing Framycetin with Hydrocortisone.

"Framyspray" (Fisons) is a pressurized spray containing Framycetin, Polymixin B and Bacitracin Zinc.

"Soframycin" (Roussel) is available as an Ointment or as a Cream containing Framycitin and Gramicidin.

"Sofracort Metred Skin Spray" (Roussel) delivers measured doses of aerosol containing Framycetin, Gramicidin and hydrocortisone.

"Sofra-Tulle" (Roussel) is a sterile paraffin gauze impregnated with Framycetin.

Nystatin B.P. is a fungistatic and fungicidal antibiotic active against *Candida* and other yeasts. It is not used against the common dermatophytes.

Pecilocin is fungistatic and inhibits the growth of *Epidermophyton, Microsporum* and *Trichophyton*. It is not effective against *Candida*.

"Variotin Ointment" (Leo Laboratories) contains Pecilocin in a neutral ointment basis.

Sodium Fusidate B.P. is the hemihydrate of the sodium salt of fusidic acid. It is a white powder very soluble in water and alcohol. It is very active against Gram-positive bacteria and Gram-negative cocci.

"Fucidin" (Leo Laboratories) is available as an ointment containing 2 per cent Sodium Fusidate.

BACITRACIN (see Antibiotics)

BENZALKONIUM CHLORIDE

Benzalkonium Chloride Solution (*Liquor Benzalkonii*) B.P. Trade names: "Roccal" (Bayer Products), "Zephiran" in U.S.A., is a mixture of alkylbenzyldimethylammonium chlorides, the alkyl groups containing from 8–18 carbon atoms. The solution contains 50 per cent w/v of Benzalkonium Chloride. It is a clear, colourless or pale yellow liquid which is miscible with water, alcohol and acetone.

Benzalkonium chloride is a cationic detergent and is therefore incompatible with soaps and other cationic detergents. It is also incompatible with nitrates, maleates, iodides, mercuric chloride, permanganates, salicylates and alkalis. Solutions should be stored in dark-coloured bottles.

A 1:1,000 solution may be used as a pre-operative detergent, but if the feet have been recently washed with soap a preliminary rinse with plain water will be required. Benzalkonium chloride possesses bactericidal properties against both Gram-positive and Gram-negative organisms and a 1:2,000 solution may be used as a wound dressing, but it loses its bactericidal properties when brought into contact with cotton or cellulose fibre. Gauze dressings must not be used. Benzalkonium chloride is not effective for sterilizing instruments but sterile instruments may be stored in a 1:4,000 solution to which sodium nitrite has been added. The continuous use of Benzalkonium Chloride Solution may cause defatting of the skin, which should be remedied by means of a suitable emollient.

"Calaxin" Cream and Powder (Calmic) each contain 0·1 per cent of Benzalkonium Chloride.

"Drapolene Cream" (Calmic) contains 0·01 per cent Benzalkonium Chloride in a water-miscible basis.

BENZOCAINE

Benzocaine (*Benzocaina*) B.P. is ethyl *p*-amino benzoate:

$$H_2N-\!\!\!\bigcirc\!\!\!-CO\cdot O\cdot C_6H_5$$

a white crystalline powder with a slightly bitter taste. It is soluble 1 part in 2,500 parts of water, 1 in 8 of alcohol 90 per cent and 1 in 4 of ether.

Benzocaine is a good surface analgesic when the skin is broken but is not very efficient on unbroken skin, because it is effective only when it is in contact with the nerve endings.

Compound Benzocaine Ointment (*Unguentum Benzocainae Compositum*) B.P.C. contains Benzocaine 10 per cent, Hamamelis Ointment 45 per cent, and Zinc Oxide Ointment 45 per cent. An alternative (unofficial) ointment is Benzocaine 10 per cent, Resorcin 2 per cent, Zinc Oxide 10 per cent, Arachis Oil 10 per cent in Hydrous Lanolin to 100 per cent.

The above ointment may be used as an antipruritic dressing for chilblains and to relieve pain in neurovascular corns. In the latter case the ointment is used as a buffer ointment in a cavity pad.

The preparation: Benzocaine 10 per cent, Tannic acid 20 per cent in Alcohol (90 per cent) may be employed as a stypic. The benzocaine stops the stinging effect of the tannic acid and the spirit.

Proprietary products were formerly sold in Great Britain under the name "Anaesthesin" (Bayer Products).

"Calobalm" (Christie, George) is a cream containing 4 per cent of Benzocaine, 0·1 per cent Aminacrine Hydrochloride and 10 per cent Calamine in an oil-in-water emulsion basic.

"Nestosyl" (Bengue) Oily solution contains benzocaine and butyl aminobenzoate. "Nestosyl" Aerosol contains 4 per cent Benzocaine, 6 per cent Butyl aminobenzoate with Hexachlorophane.

"Intralgin" (Riker) is an application for strains, sprains and unbroken chilblains containing 1·86 per cent of Benzocaine, 4·65 per cent of Salicylamide and Isopropyl Alcohol 60 per cent.

"Polycrest Cream" (Nicholas Laboratories) contains 5 per cent Benzocaine, 0·25 per cent Phenylmercuric Nitrate and 0·5 per cent Amethocaine Hydrochloride in a non-greasy base.

BENZOIC ACID

Benzoic Acid (*Acidum Benzoicum*) B.P. consists of white feathery crystals containing at least 99·5 per cent of $C_6H_5 \cdot COOH$. Benzoic Acid is a preservative and mild antiseptic, and is present in Benzoin, Storax, and the Balsams of Peru and Tolu.

Benzoic Acid is incompatible with ferric salts, including ferric chloride and with mercuric chloride.

Compound Benzoic Acid Ointment (*Unguentum Acidi Benzoici Compositum*) B.P.C. syn. Whitfield's Ointment.

Whitfield's Ointment contains Benzoic Acid 6 per cent, Salicylic Acid 3 per cent in Emulsifying Ointment to 100 per cent.

N.B. Whitfield's Ointment in the B.P.C., 1949, contained 5 per cent (not 6 per cent) of Benzoic Acid. Whitfield's original formula was: Benzoic Acid 5 per cent, Salicylic Acid 3 per cent in Soft Paraffin 25 per cent and Coconut Oil to 100 per cent.

Whitfield's Ointment is indicated in the treatment of dermatomycosis and in cases where mycotic infection is suspected as a complication of fissures, soft corns or plaster dermatitis. Benzoic acid is not in itself keratolytic, but in Whitfield's Ointment it so enhances the action of the salicylic acid that the effect of the combination is to destroy the horny layer of the skin. Because the horny layer is destroyed, the treatment of dermatomycosis with Whitfield's Ointment is better adapted to hospital than to ambulatory treatment. Nevertheless, it is a very effective treatment where it can be adapted to suit the needs of chiropody. The ointment should be rubbed into the mycotic lesions daily by the patient.

BENZOIN

Benzoin (*Benzoinum*) B.P.C. is a balsamic resin from *Styrax benzoin* or *Styrax paralleloneurus* and contains 30–60 per cent of free balsamic acids.

Benzoin Tincture (*Tinctura Benzoini*) B.P.C. consists of 10 parts of Benzoin in 90 parts of 90 per cent Alcohol and is sometimes used in lieu of the more usual Compound Benzoin Tincture.

Compound Benzoin Tincture (*Tinctura Benzoini Composita*) B.P.C. syn. Friars' Balsam, contains Benzoin 10 per cent, prepared Storax 7·5 per cent, Tolu Balsam 2·5 per cent, Aloes 2 per cent in 90 per cent, Alcohol to 100 per cent.

Compound Benzoin Tincture (*Methylated*) is prepared with I.M.S. instead of 90 per cent alcohol. This preparation is considerably cheaper than the B.P. preparation to which it is similar, except that it can be used only externally. It is to be recommended for use by chiropodists.

Compound Benzoin Tincture is incompatible with water until the tincture has dried out due to the evaporation of the alcohol. Bottles which have contained Friars' Balsam should always be cleaned with alcohol, and Friars' Balsam should never be poured away down a sink because the precipitated resins may block the pipes. Compound Benzoin Tincture is slightly astringent, it is antiseptic on the intact skin and, due to the aloe content, is mildly styptic. It promotes healthy granulation of minor wounds and abrasions. When it is applied to the skin and allowed to dry, it forms an occlusive film over the skin surface and is therefore contra-indicated in pustular and weeping conditions.

Compound Benzoin Tincture may be used in the following ways:

1. As a routine dressing, applied as a paint after operating. It affords some protection to the skin from the effects of rubber adhesive and also prevents the rapid hardening of callus due to "drying-out".

2. As a daily paint to chilblains, either alone, or half and half with Weak Iodine Solution or Strong Iodine Solution.

3. As a daily application to fissures: 3—5 per cent of Salicylic Acid may be incorporated in the Compound Benzoin Tincture if the complication of mycotic infection is suspected.

4. When the skin has suffered mechanical abrasion due to the application of rubber adhesive, a painting of Compound Benzoin Tincture forms an antiseptic and protective layer on the surface. Several layers of the tincture may be used, each layer being allowed to dry before the next is applied. This method gives protection when the skin is showing a mild reaction to rubber adhesive.

The tincture needs to have dried somewhat before adhesive materials can be applied to the skin, but as the tincture dries after a minute or two it becomes tacky and helps with close adhesion of the protective materials. The use of a dusting powder counteracts any residual tackiness and prevents the stocking from sticking to the foot.

5. To assist operating on soft corns, because it supplies the knife with some grip on slippery tissues.

6. As an application with a pack for a nail groove: the Compound Tincture helps the pack to adhere to the nail groove and makes it more resistant to water. It makes a somewhat hard and stiff dressing.

7. As a protection to the skin, when applying an acid ointment in the treatment of warts, etc. The tissues round the lesion may be

painted with several layers of Compound Benzoin Tincture, the lesion itself being left uncovered.

"Rikospray Balsam" (Riker) is an aerosol spray solution containing soluble benzoic solids 9 per cent (equivalent to Benzoin 12 per cent) and Prepared Storax 2·5 per cent with solvent and propellant.

BORIC ACID

Boric Acid (*Acidum Boricum*) B.P. syn. Boracic Acid occurs as colourless unctuous scales or crystals, or as a white powder containing not less than 99·5 per cent of H_3BO_3. It has a bitter taste. Boric acid is soluble 1 part in 20 parts of water, 1 in 3 of boiling water, 1 in 18 of alcohol and 1 in 4 of glycerin.

Boric acid is incompatible with tannin.

Boric acid inhibits bacterial growth but is toxic when absorbed by the tissues. Because it is readily absorbed from dressings such preparations as Boric Acid Gauze were popular. It must not be thought, however, that a dry dressing of Boric Acid Gauze gives sufficient protection when a haemorrhage has occurred. Boric acid is said to have a specific action on the organisms responsible for the breakdown of sweat in certain cases of bromidrosis and was therefore widely used as an ingredient of dusting-powders. Because it is toxic when absorbed, Boric acid preparations should be used with great caution. Boric Acid Ointment, because of its slight antiseptic quality and its stiff base, may be used as a buffer in cavity pads. Boric Acid Ointment is contra-indicated as a dressing following the breakdown of warts which have been treated with acids.

Boric Acid Gauze (*Carbasus Acidi Borici*) B.P.C. 1954 contains 3–7 per cent of Boric Acid.

Boric Acid Lint (*Linteum Acidi Borici*) B.P.C. contains 3–7 per cent of Boric Acid.

Boric Acid Ointment (*Unguentum Acidi Borici*) B.P.C. contains 1 per cent of Boric Acid in Paraffin Ointment 99 per cent.

Boric Talc Dusting-powder (*Conspersus Talci Borici*) B.P.C. 1963 contains 5 per cent of Boric Acid, 10 per cent of Starch and 85 per cent of Purified Talc.

Compound Salicylic Acid Dusting-powder (*Conspersus Acidi Salicylici Compositus*) B.P.C. 1963 syn. Pulvis pro Pedibus contains 3 per cent of Salicylic Acid, 5 per cent of Boric Acid and 92 per cent of Purified Talc.

Compound Zinc Dusting-powder (*Conspersus Zinci Compositus*) B.P.C. 1963 contains 5 per cent of Boric Acid, 25 per cent Zinc Oxide, 35 per cent Starch and 35 per cent Talc.

Dusting-powders containing more than 5 per cent of Boric Acid should be labelled: "Not to be applied to raw or weeping surfaces".

BRILLIANT GREEN

Brilliant Green (*Viride Nitens*) B.P. is Anhydrodi (*p*-diethylamino) triphenylmethanol hydrogen sulphate. It occurs as small green crystals which are soluble in water giving a green solution. Like crystal violet, brilliant green is derived from triphenylmethane.

Unlike crystal violet, brilliant green is effective against the Coli-typhoid group of organisms and is effective against Gram-negative organisms. It is frequently used on septic lesions if the discharge is thin and watery, indicating the possibility of infection with strepto-cocci or with Gram-negative organisms. Brilliant green is employed as a wound dressing as a 1:1,000 aqueous solution or as a 2 per cent ointment. Brilliant green stimulates healthy epithelialization and is therefore useful in the treatment of indolent ulcers.

Brilliant green is often employed in mixtures with crystal violet and proflavine. In combination, the dyes are effective against a wider range of organisms than they are when used individually.

Brilliant Green and Crystal Violet Paint (*Pigmentum Tinctorum*) B.P.C. 1954 contains 0·5 per cent of Brilliant Green, 0·5 per cent of Crystal Violet, 50 per cent of Alcohol (90 per cent) with water to 100 per cent.

Compound Crystal Violet Paint (*Pigmentum Violae Crystallinae Compositum*) B.P.C. 1954 contains 0·229 per cent of Crystal Violet, 0·229 per cent of Brilliant Green, 0·114 per cent of Proflavine Hemi-sulphate in water to 100 per cent.

Malachite Green is sometimes used in lieu of Brilliant Green. A 2 per cent solution of malachite green in spirit will reduce hyper-granulation tissue and is particularly valuable in dealing with proud flesh associated with onychocryptosis.

CALAMINE

Calamine (*Calamina*) B.P. is a basic zinc carbonate, with or without zinc oxide, yielding 68–74 per cent of zinc oxide on ignition. It is coloured pink with ferric oxide. In appearance calamine is a heavy pink powder which is insoluble in water and alcohol, but which is soluble (with effervescence) in acids.

Calamine is soothing, astringent and absorbent; it will absorb about one and a half times its own weight of moisture.

Compound Calamine Application (*Applicatio Calaminae Composita*) B.P.C. contains 10 per cent of Calamine, 5 per cent of Zinc Oxide in a Cream prepared with Zinc Stearate, Wool Fat, White Soft Paraffin and Liquid Paraffin.

Compound Calamine Application is indicated in itching or weeping skin conditions or for mild plaster dermatitis. The cream is painted on and generally no dressings are applied.

Calamine Lotion (Lotio Calaminae) B.P. contains 15 per cent of Calamine, 5 per cent of Zinc Oxide, 3 per cent of Bentonite, 0·5 of Phenol, 5 per cent of Glycerin and 0·5 per cent of Sodium Citrate in Distilled Water to 100 per cent.

Oily Calamine Lotion (Lotio Calaminae Oleosa) B.P.C. syn. Liniment of Calamine, contains 5 per cent of Calamine, 1 per cent of Wool Fat, 0·5 per cent of Oleic Acid, 50 per cent of Arachis Oil in Solution of Calcium Hydroxide to 100 per cent.

The Lotions of Calamine are indicated for pruritic skin conditions, plaster rash and chilblains to relieve itching. They are painted on and allowed to dry.

Calamine Ointment (Unguentum Calaminae) B.P.C. contains Calamine 15·0 per cent and White Soft Paraffin 85·0 per cent.

"Dermogesic Ointment" (Sharpe & Dohme) contains Calamine 8 per cent, Benzocaine 3 per cent, Hexylated m-cresol 0·05 per cent in a vanishing cream base.

"Lacto-Calamine" (Crookes) incorporates 11·5 per cent of a colloidal processed Calamine with Witch Hazel in a soothing lotion base.

"Lacto-Calamine Cream" (Crookes) contains Crookes' Calamine 5 per cent with Witch Hazel in a vanishing-cream base.

"Lacto-Calamine Talcum Powder" (Crookes) contains Crookes' Calamine 5 per cent.

CALCIUM SALTS

Chalk (*Creta*) B.P. is a native calcium carbonate ($CaCo_3$) purified by elutriation and containing not less than 97 per cent of $CaCO_3$. (N.B. Calcium Carbonate B.P. is prepared by the interaction of a soluble calcium salt and a soluble carbonate.) Chalk is a very fine white amorphous powder which is insoluble either in water or in alcohol.

Chalk is a lubricant, and is used as such in dusting-powders.

Calcium Hydroxide (*Calcii Hydroxidum*) B.P. ($Ca[OH]_2$) is made by the action of water on calcium oxide. It is a white powder which is more soluble in cold than in hot water.

Calcium Hydroxide Solution (*Liquor Calcii Hydroxidi*) B.P. syn. Lime Water is a saturated solution of calcium hydroxide in water.

Lime water should contain not less than 0·15 per cent of calcium hydroxide.

Lime water may be applied as an astringent lotion in skin affections for which purpose it may be combined with calamine. It counteracts excessive acidity of the skin and thus relieves itching.

Calcium Hydroxide Solution may be used in combination with a fat in the preparations of emulsions. The calcium hydroxide, acting with the fat, forms a soap, which acts as an emulsifying agent. A preparation consisting of equal parts of lime water and linseed oil is a useful treatment for burns caused by Phenol.

Dried Calcium Sulphate (*Calcii Sulphas Exsiccatus*) B.P.C. syn. Plaster of Paris, $CaSO_4, \frac{1}{2}H_2O$, is a white hygroscopic powder, which is slightly soluble in water.

A mixture of $1\frac{1}{2}$–2 parts of water to 1 part of dried calcium sulphate forms a smooth paste which sets rapidly to form a hard mass. If the exsiccated calcium sulphate has been heated to above 200° C., or if much atmospheric moisture has been absorbed it will not set. The setting time may be retarded by using a 5 per cent solution of dextrin instead of water in preparing the mix, or by adding acacia or a citrate to the powder. Setting may be accelerated by adding sodium chloride, alum or potassium sulphate to the powder. Plaster of Paris deteriorates rapidly, deterioration being shown by very quick or very slow setting and by the production of a friable or weakened mass when setting takes place. Plaster of Paris is used for making casts in the preparation of remedial appliances.

Calcium Alginate B.P.C. consists mainly of the calcium salt of alginic acid. It may contain some of the sodium salt. It occurs as a white or yellowish powder or fibres, insoluble in water and organic solvents.

Calcium alginate is used as an absorbable haemostatic. Fibres of calcium alginate are used to prepare a "gauze" and the gauze is used to cover or to pack wounds.

"Calgitex" (Medical Alginates) is a range of sterile absorbable dressings composed of calcium and sodium alginates obtainable as wool, alginate dressings for first aid, gauze and ribbon gauze.

CAMPHOR

Camphor (*Camphora*) B.P. ($C_{10}H_{16}O$) is a colourless transparent, crystalline substance obtained from the wood of a tree, *Cinnamomum camphora*. It may be prepared synthetically. It is soluble 1 part in 700 parts of water and 1 in 1 of alcohol (90 per cent).

Camphor is rubefacient, antipruritic, fungicidal and antiseptic.

When applied to the skin, it first stimulates and then numbs the peripheral sensory nerves. It gives a sense of coldness owing to an increase in the sensitivity to cold of the nerve endings in the skin.

Camphor liquefies with chloral hydrate, menthol, phenol, thymol, resorcinol, betanaphthol or pyrogallol.

Rectified Camphor Oil (*Oleum Camphorae Rectificatum*) B.P.C. 1959 is obtained in the manufacture of natural camphor and contains not less than 30 per cent of the active principle cineole. Oil of camphor may be employed as a fungicidal paint.

Camphor Liniment (*Linimentum Camphorae*) B.P. syn. Camphorated Oil consists of Camphor 20 per cent in Arachis Oil 80 per cent. This may be used as a general rubefacient.

Camphor may also be used in dusting-powders as a fungicide, and is a common ingredient of rubefacient liniments.

"Pernione Ointment" (Philip Harris) contains 2·5 per cent Camphor, 2·5 per cent Iodine, 2·5 per cent Methyl Salicylate, 2·5 per cent Ichthammol, 2·5 per cent Peru Balsam, 5 per cent Glycerin. For chilblains.

CAPSICUM

Capsicum (*Capsicum*) B.P.C. syn. Cayenne is the dried fruit of *Capsicum minimum* and contains about 0·5 to 0·9 per cent of capsaicin.

Applied externally capsicum is a very active rubefacient.

Capsicum Ointment (*Unguentum Capsici*) B.P.C. contains 250 grammes of Capsicum in 950 grammes of Simple Ointment. This is strongly rubefacient ointment, which may be applied in certain cases of chilblains and for neuralgic conditions.

Capsicum Cotton Wool (*Gossypium Capsici*) B.P.C. is absorbent cotton wool impregnated with the Oleoresin of Capsicum and with Methyl Salicylate. It is tinted orange-brown.

Gauze and Capsicum Cotton Tissue (*Tela Carbasi et Gossypii Capsici*) B.P.C. Trade names: "Thermogene" (Veno Drug Co.), "Capsogen" (Southall) consists of Capsicum Cotton Wool in absorbent gauze.

The above two preparations may be applied externally as rubefacients. Their rubefacient action is enhanced because the heat brought about by the hyperaemia, produced by their use, is conserved by the insulating action of the cotton wool which prevents loss of heat by radiation.

"Capsolin" (Parke Davis) contains Oleoresin of Capsicum 13 minims, Camphor 23 grains, Oil of Turpentine 13½ minims, Oil of Eucalyptus 13 minims, base to one ounce.

CARBON DIOXIDE

Carbon dioxide may be used in chiropody for two widely differing purposes.

1. *As a Carbon Dioxide Foot-bath.* A warm Carbon Dioxide foot-bath is particularly useful in the relief of congestion in a limb or foot, and may be used also in cases of sepsis.

Sodium bicarbonate powder is dissolved in a foot-bath containing about 10 litres (two gallons) of water at 50° C. (112° F.). The foot or limb is then immersed in the water and a few crystals of tartaric acid are added. The sodium bicarbonate and the tartaric acid interact to liberate CO_2. In cases of sepsis an antiseptic such as "Hibitane" or "Dettol" may be added to the water, and the crystals may be so placed in the water as to direct the stream of carbon dioxide bubbles at the septic cavity.

A close approximation to *Effervescent Bath* (*Balneum Effervescens*) B.P.C. 1949 may be prepared by dissolving 15 grammes (half an ounce) of Sodium Bicarbonate in 5 litres (one gallon) of warm water and adding 7·5 grammes of Sodium Acid Sulphate. Similarly a close approximation of *Saline Effervescent Bath* (*Balneum Effervescens cum Chloridis*) B.P.C. 1949 may be prepared by dissolving in 5 litres (one gallon) of warm water 15 grammes (half an ounce) of Sodium Bicarbonate, 7·5 grammes of Calcium Chloride and adding 7·5 grammes (quarter of an ounce) of Sodium Acid Sulphate. These ingredients are also found in "Nauheim Bath Salts".

N.B. Some operators use hydrochloric acid in place of tartaric acid in the first method. In this case 25 ml. of concentrated hydrochloric acid is added to 5 litres of water, and crystals of sodium bicarbonate are added in order to produce effervescence. This is the only purpose for which concentrated hydrochloric acid is used in chiropody and the acid is dangerous unless it is carefully handled. There is no advantage in using hydrochloric acid but the liability to accidents is increased.

2. *As Carbon Dioxide Snow in the treatment of warts.* The method used is as follows:

(i) Remove the superficial layers of the wart.

(ii) The carbon dioxide snow is prepared in accordance with the instructions supplied with the particular form of apparatus which is being used.

(iii) The end of the "pencil" is cut to the size and shape of the wart.

(iv) The predetermined dose is administered to the wart. The dosage varies according to the time of application and the amount of pressure used. Sixty seconds of moderate pressure is an average dose.

(v) The foot is placed in a warm foot-bath for about 5 minutes. This procedure obviates much of the pain which may be experienced when carbon dioxide snow is used.

(vi) The wart is dressed in the usual way with a dressing of 60 per cent salicylic acid ointment. The return period is 5–7 days. A more active reaction to the salicylic acid than is usual is to be expected.

Steps (v) and (vi) may be omitted. If they are left out, a blister should have formed when the patient returns. The contents of the blister should be evacuated and the blister dressed with an antiseptic dressing (*not* Cream of Proflavine). Whitfield recommended soaking the growth with water prior to applying the snow. The saturated tissues transmit the cold more readily and a deeper penetration results.

The use of carbon dioxide snow on warts is indicated in deep single growths which have proved resistant to other types of treatment.

CARBON TETRACHLORIDE

Carbon Tetrachloride (*Carbonei Tetrachloridum*) B.P. is tetrachloromethane (CCl_4). It is a heavy, colourless, volatile liquid with a characteristic odour.

Carbon tetrachloride is used in chiropody as a solvent for the pre-operative preparation of the skin. It is rather less popular than acetone and ether as a pre-operative solvent, but it has the great advantage of being non-inflammable. The fumes of carbon tetrachloride are poisonous in moderate concentrations, and it must be used with great care. Carbon tetrachloride does not readily dissolve certain brands of rubber adhesive plaster but, with other brands, it is as effective as ether. Because it is less volatile it is more effective than ether in removing fresh plaster marks from the skin. It is contraindicated for general use and should be reserved for occasional use when other solvents will not act.

"Thawpit" (Thawpit, Ltd.) is pure Carbon Tetrachloride.

"Zoff" (Smith & Nephew) is an adhesive plaster remover. It is non-inflammable.

CASTOR OIL (see Oils, Expressed)

CETOSTEARYL ALCOHOL (see Alcohols)

CETRIMIDE

Cetrimide (*Cetrimidum*) B.P. syn. C.T.A.B. Trade names: "Cetavlon" (I.C.I. Pharmaceuticals), "Biocetab" (Biorex) consists of a mixture of dodecyl-, tetradecyl- and hexadecyl-trimethylammonium bromides (see also page 35), and contains 98–102 per cent of alkyl trimethyl ammonium bromides calculated as $C_{17}H_{38}NBr$. Cetrimide is a creamy-white unctuous powder which is soluble one part in two of water and is readily soluble in alcohol. It is sometimes difficult to dissolve cetrimide in tap water and, wherever possible, distilled water should be used for preparing solutions. It should *not* be stored in *corked* bottles.

A solution of cetrimide in water reduces the surface tension of the water which readily forms a foam. Cetrimide is a cationic detergent, the water-soluble portion of the molecule carrying a negative charge, and it is therefore incompatible with soap and with other anionic detergents. It is also incompatible with iodine, phenylmercuric nitrate, phenol, chlorocresol and alkali hydroxides.

Cetrimide has two distinct actions:
1. It is a detergent.
2. It is a bactericide.

As a bactericide cetrimide is effective in concentrations of about 0·1 per cent and is active against both Gram-positive and Gram-negative organisms. In concentrations of 1 per cent or over cetrimide acts as a detergent and a 1 per cent solution is active both as a detergent and as a bactericide. When it is used as a detergent the solution of cetrimide must be removed after application, either with a swab of cotton wool or, preferably, by rinsing with water so that it carries away with it the dirt and grease from the skin. If cetrimide is used as a bactericide it is applied as a wet dressing and allowed to remain in contact with the bacteria for a considerable period of time. It kills the bacteria which remain *in situ*. Cetrimide is a very efficient detergent and it may remove much of the natural grease from the operator's hands and from the patient's feet and thus reduce the natural resistance of the skin. For pre-operative preparation of the skin, it is suggested that a 1 per cent solution should be used as a detergent and followed by a paint of 0·1 per cent solution which should be allowed to dry on the skin. If cetrimide solution is not used as a detergent before applying the paint, the former, in order to be effective, must be in contact with the bacteria for an appreciable time. For instance, a 0·1 per cent solution in 70 per cent alcohol must be left on the skin for at least two minutes and a 10 per cent solution in 70 per cent alcohol for at least half a minute.

A 1 per cent solution of cetrimide is sometimes used for sterilizing instruments; 0·2 per cent of sodium nitrite should be added to the solution to prevent rusting. It must be remembered that cetrimide, being a detergent, will remove the protective film of grease which is normally present on all instruments and that therefore instruments which have been immersed in a cetrimide solution will tend to corrode rapidly at the cutting edge when they are removed from it.

Solutions of cetrimide in strengths from 0·1–1 per cent may also be used as post-operative antiseptics on broken or unbroken skin.

Cetrimide Cream (*Cremor Cetrimidi*) B.P.C. contains 0·5 per cent of Cetrimide in a cream base. Store in a cool place.

Cetrimide Solution (*Liquor Cetrimidi*) B.P.C. is a 2·5 per cent aqueous solution of Cetrimide. It must be used within 7 days of preparation. Cork closures must not be used.

Strong Cetrimide Solution B.P.C. is a 40 per cent solution of Cetrimide in water with 7·5 per cent v/v of alcohol. The solution must not come into contact with cork.

"Gomaxine Antiseptic Cream" (Riddell) contains 0·5 per cent of Cetrimide.

"Cetavlex Cream" (I.C.I.) contains 0·5 per cent of Cetrimide in a water-miscible basis.

"Savlon Cream" (I.C.I.) is an antiseptic cream containing 0·5 per cent of Cetrimide.

"Savlon Liquid Antiseptic" (I.C.I.) contains Cetrimide 3 per cent and Chlorhexidine Gluconate 0·3 per cent and is a general and domestic disinfectant.

"Savlon Hospital Concentrate" (I.C.I.) contains 15 per cent of Cetrimide and Chlorhexidine gluconate 1·5 per cent.

"Vesagex" (Willows Francis) is a non-greasy ointment containing 1·0 per cent of Cetrimide.

"Tred" (Priory Laboratories) is an ointment containing 1·5 per cent of Cetrimide.

"Cetavlon Concentrate" (I.C.I.) 40 per cent or 20 per cent solutions of Cetrimide used to prepare dilute solutions.

CHALK (see Calcium Salts)

CHLORAL HYDRATE, CHLORBUTOL

Chloral Hydrate (*Chloralis Hydras*) B.P. is trichlorethylidene glycol $CCl_3 \cdot CH(OH)_2$. It occurs as colourless crystals containing not less than 99·0 per cent of $C_2H_3O_2Cl_3$. Chloral hydrate is soluble in water, alcohol and glycerin.

Chloral hydrate is incompatible with alkalis, ammonium salts, borax, tannin, potassium iodide and potassium permanganate.

Chloral hydrate is antiseptic, analgesic and antipruritic in strengths from 1–5 per cent. Above 5 per cent it is a rubefacient and in high strengths it is caustic.

Chloral hydrate up to 5 per cent strength may be employed as an ingredient in ointments for the treatment of the hyperaemic stage of chilblains. Up to 5 per cent of chloral hydrate may be incorporated as an analgesic, in caustic ointments of salicylic acid.

Chlorbutol (*Chlorbutol*) B.P. is 2, 2, 2-Trichloro-1, 1-dimethyl-ethanol hemihydrate, $CCl_3 \cdot C(CH_3)_2 \cdot OH$. It occurs as colourless crystals containing not less than 93 per cent of $C_4H_7OCl_3$. Chlorbutol is antiseptic and fungicidal. It is also an antipruritic. It may be used as an ingredient of dusting-powders in a strength of 1 or 2 per cent.

"Mycozol" (Parke, Davis) Ointment contains 5 per cent of Chlorbutol, 4 per cent of Salicylic Acid and 4 per cent of Mercury Salicylate. "Mycozol" Dusting-powder contains Chlorbutol 5 per cent, Salicylic Acid 2 per cent, Mercury Salicylate 4 per cent in a Starch and Talc basis. For fungal infections of the skin.

"Mycozol Liquid" contains 5 per cent of Chlorbutol, 2 per cent of Salicylic Acid, 2 per cent of Benzoic Acid and 0·1 per cent of Malachite Green. It is a fungicide.

CHLORAMINE (see Chlorine)

CHLORINE—INORGANIC AND ORGANIC PREPARATIONS

Chlorinated Lime (*Calx Chlorinata*) B.P. syn. Bleaching Powder contains not less than 30 per cent of available chlorine. It may, on occasions, be used to remove dyes from the skin and when it is used for this purpose it should be followed by a rinse of 10 per cent solution of sodium metabisulphide and a further rinse in plain water.

Chlorinated Lime and Boric Acid Solution (*Liquor Calcis Chlorinae et Acidi Borici* B.P.C. syn. Eusol is a solution of 1·25 per cent of Chlorinated Lime and 1·25 per cent of Boric Acid in water.

This solution, which should be freshly prepared, was formerly much used in the treatment of septic wounds. It is applied as a wet dressing without waterproof cover.

Surgical Chlorinated Soda Solution (*Liquor Sodae Chlorinatae Chirugicalis*) B.P.C. syn. Dakin's Solution is prepared from Chlorinated Lime, Sodium Carbonate and Boric Acid. It contains from 0·5–0·55 per cent of available chlorine. Dakin's Solution should be stored away from the light and in a cool place.

Dakin's solution is a non-irritating antiseptic for wounds, especially septic wounds. Fresh solution should be brought into contact with the wounds by frequent changes of dressing. Dakin's solution aids the dissolution of necrosed tissue by forming stable chloramines.

As a class, the chlorine antiseptics probably exert a physiological rather than a direct antiseptic action, in that they stimulate the flow of tissue fluid. The inorganic chlorine antiseptics are now less frequently used than formerly, although the electrolytically prepared hypochlorites retain a place in the field of antiseptics. The hypochlorites are frequently used for the sterilization of equipment and kitchen utensils.

Proprietary products containing hypochlorites include: "Chloros" (I.C.I.), "Deosan Green Label" and "Diversol BX" (Diversey), "Hyposan" and "Voxsan" (Voxsan Ltd.) and "Milton Antiseptic" (Vick International).

Chloramine (*Chloraimina*) B.P.C. is toluene-*p*-sulphonsodiochloroamide. It occurs as white crystals or powder soluble in water and alcohol.

Chloramine is incompatible with alcohol, hydrogen peroxide and should not be used with other antiseptics. Solutions should be freshly prepared.

Chloramine may be used as a 2 per cent solution in water for the treatment of infected wounds, in lieu of Dakin's solution. It is non-irritant and practically non-toxic.

"Dygerma" (Matthews Laboratories) is a stabilized solution of chloramines, 5 per cent used as a general antiseptic.

Chloroazodin B.P.C. 1949. Trade name: "Azochloramid" may be used in lieu of Chloramine.

Chlorphenesin B.P. is 3-*p*-Chlorophenoxypropane-1,-2 diol. Cl·C_6H_4·OCH_2·CHOH·CH_2OH. It is a powerful fungicide and is especially useful in resistant cases.

Chlorphenesin Dusting-powder B.P.C. contains 1 per cent Chlorphenesin, 18 per cent Talc, 25 per cent Zinc Oxide and 56 per cent Starch.

"Mycil" (B.D.H.) is Chlorphenesin available as a 0·5 per cent ointment, a 1 per cent powder and a 1 per cent aerosol spray.

There is a number of antimycotic drugs which are organic chlorine compounds. They include:

"Asterol" (Roche) Diamethazole hydrochloride available as Ointment, Dusting-powder or Tincture, each containing 5 per cent.

"S7" (Calmic) Fenticlor as a 1 per cent Cream, Jelly or Powder.

"Tinaderm" (Glaxo) Dusting-powder contains 1 per cent Tolnaftate.

"Episol" (Crookes) Halethazole 0·5 per cent as a Lotion, Cream or Dusting-powder.

"Jadit" (Hoechst) Buclosamide available as an Ointment, 10 per cent with 2 per cent Salicylic Acid, or as a Powder or Solution each containing 10 per cent with 1 per cent Salicylic Acid.

CHLORHEXIDINE (see Halogenated Phenols)

CHLOROAZODIN (see Chlorine)

CHLOROCRESOL (see Halogenated Phenols)

CHLOROXYLENOL (see Halogenated Phenols)

CHLORPHENESIN (see Chlorine)

CLIOQUINOL (see Iodine)

CLOVE OIL (see Oils, Essential)

COAL TAR

Prepared Coal Tar (*Pix Carbonis Preparata*) B.P.C. is commercial coal tar heated to 50° C. for 1 hour. It is a black liquid having a strong characteristic odour.

Coal tar is antiseptic, antipruritic, stimulating and is mildly rubefacient. It is sometimes incorporated with calamine preparations. Coal tar preparations are indicated in cases of psoriasis, eczema and broken and unbroken chilblains.

Coal Tar Solution (*Liquor Picis Carbonis*) B.P. contains Prepared Coal Tar 20 per cent, Quillaia 10 per cent, (90 per cent) Alcohol 70 per cent.

Coal Tar Paste (*Pasta Picis Carbonis*) B.P.C. contains 7·5 per cent of Strong Coal Tar Solution with Compound Paste of Zinc Oxide to 100 per cent.

Calamine and Coal Tar Ointment (*Unguentum Calaminae et Picis Carbonis*) B.P.C. contains 12·5 per cent of Calamine, 12·5 per cent of Zinc Oxide, 2·5 per cent of Strong Coal Tar Solution, 25 per cent of Hydrous Wool Fat with White Soft Paraffin to 100 per cent.

"E.S.T.P." (Martindale) Ether-soluble Tar Paste is a bland and soothing ointment for the treatment of skin conditions.

"Tar Dermament" (Parke, Davis) contains the equivalent of 6 per cent washed Coal Tar combined with alcohol-soluble phenolic resin which remains on the skin after drying and forms upon it a protective water-resistant film. It is particularly useful where two skin surfaces are in apposition.

COD-LIVER OIL

Cod Liver Oil (*Oleum Morrhuae*) B.P. is expressed from the fresh liver of the cod, *Gadus callarias*, and is freed from fat by filtration at 0° C. It is a pale yellow liquid with a slightly fishy odour and taste.

The main use of cod-liver oil is internally, as a source of vitamins A and D. Incorporated in Creams and Ointments cod-liver oil promotes healthy granulation and also has an emollient effect. One part of cod-liver oil may be mixed with 9 parts of olive oil, 3 parts of lanolin and 3 parts of soft paraffin to give a rather greasy emollient.

"Bornolin" (Bengue & Co.) contains Cod-liver Oil, Halibut-liver Oil and Vitamin D in Yellow Soft Paraffin. This is recommended for the treatment of scalds, burns and septic wounds. It is applied on lint and the dressing should be renewed every two days.

"Morhulin Ointment" (Priory Laboratories) contains chlorinated Cod-liver Oil 11·4 per cent, Zinc Oxide 38 per cent, Wool Fat 10 per cent in Soft Paraffin to 100 per cent.

"Morhulin Powder" contains 4·5 per cent of Cod-liver Oil, with Balsam of Peru, Zinc Oxide, Boric Acid, Talc and Kaolin.

"Morhulinol" is an ointment containing chlorinated Cod-liver Oil 19·5 per cent in Balsam of Peru and Yellow Soft Paraffin.

Cod-liver Oil is an ingredient of "W.P. Ointment" ("Wheat Germ & Pyrogallol Ointment"). The ointment contains Pyrogallol 20 per cent, Wheat Germ Oil 20 per cent, Hard Paraffin 20 per cent, Hydrous Lanolin 30 per cent and Cod-liver Oil 10 per cent.

COLLODION (see Pyroxylin)

COLOPHONY

Colophony (*Colophonium*) B.P. syn. Resin, Rosin is the residue left after distilling the volatile oil of turpentine from the oleoresin of various species of pine (*Pinus*). It is a glassy, pale yellow, sticky powder.

Colophony may be used to aid the mechanical reduction of onychogryphosis with the nail drill. The powder is sprinkled on to the nail before using the drill. Colophony may also be used as an ingredient in the base of salicylic acid ointments.

Colophony Ointment (*Unguentum Colophonii*) B.P.C. 1959 syn. Basilicon Ointment contains Colophony 26 per cent, Yellow Beeswax 26 per cent, Olive Oil 26 per cent and Lard 22 per cent. Basilicon ointment is indicated as an application to ulcers and septic wounds and it tends to bring incipient sepsis to a head. It is protective and a gentle stimulant.

Lead with Colophony Plaster-mass (*Emplastrum Plumbi cum Colophonio in Massa*) B.P.C. 1954 contains Colophony 10 per cent, Plaster-mass of Lead 85 per cent with Hard Soap 5 per cent.

Lead with Soap Plaster-mass (*Emplastrum Plumbi cum Sapone in Massa*) B.P.C. 1954 contains 2·5 per cent of Colophony, 14 per cent of Hard Soap and 83·5 per cent of Plaster-mass of Lead.

COPPER SULPHATE

Copper Sulphate (*Cupri Sulphas*) B.P.C. contains not less than 98·5 per cent of $CuSO_4·5H_2O$. It occurs as blue crystals which are soluble in water but insoluble in alcohol.

Copper sulphate is astringent or caustic, and fungicidal.

A moistened crystal of copper sulphate may be rubbed into hypergranulation tissue (R.P. 4–10 days). This treatment may be carried out daily at home by a reliable patient. A saturated solution of copper sulphate may be applied once daily for 1 week to vascular corns. At the end of the week the patient should return for treatment in the surgery.

Copper and Zinc Sulphates Lotion (*Lotio Cupri et Zinci Sulphatum*) B.P.C. syn. Lotio D'Alibour, Dalibour Water contains 1·0 per cent Copper Sulphate, 1·5 per cent of Zinc Sulphate in Camphor Water to 100 per cent. This is an astringent and fungicidal lotion for the treatment of weeping skin conditions, and especially for plaster dermatitis with an underlying fungal infection.

Copper sulphate is an ingredient in "Clinitest" (Ames), a proprietary diagnostic test supplied with a colour chart, for the detection and estimation of sugar in the urine.

CREOSOTE

Creosote (*Creosotum*) B.P.C. 1959 is a mixture of phenols, chiefly guaiacol and cresol. It is a pale yellow liquid with a characteristic odour. It is soluble 1 part in 150 parts of water and is miscible with alcohol and ether.

Creosote is analgesic, antiseptic and fungicidal and is used extensively as an analgesic in proprietary corn paints, replacing *cannabis indica* which was formerly used. An ointment containing 10 per cent of creosote may be used in the treatment of mycotic skin infections.

CRESOL

Cresol (*Cresol*) B.P. is a yellowish liquid with a tar-like odour and is a mixture of three isomers corresponding to the formula $C_6H_4\cdot CH_3OH$. The isomers differ in the relative positions of the methyl (CH_3) and hydroxyl (OH) groups in the benzene ring thus:

*ortho*cresol   *meta*cresol   *para*cresol
o-cresol   *m*-cresol   *p*-cresol

Cresol is soluble 1 part in 50 parts of water and is more readily soluble in soap solutions. It is soluble also in alcohol, ether and glycerin.

Cresol Solution and Soap (*Liquor Cresolis Saponatus*) B.P. syn. Lysol, may be produced by any method so long as the final product contains 50 per cent v/v of cresols in a saponaceous solvent. Usually linseed oil or castor oil soap is used.

Lysol is a powerful germicide. Its activity is decreased by the presence of organic material. Pure Lysol has been used for instrument sterilization and a 1–2 per cent solution has been used in the instrument tray. Lysol is highly caustic and its use has been almost completely replaced by the halogenated phenols of which there is a wide selection (see page 176).

Solution of Cresol with Soap is marketed under various names including: "Acrosyl" (Monsanto), "Jeysol" (Jeyes), "Kymol" (Newton Chambers) and "Lysol" (Marshall's Lysol).

CRYSTAL VIOLET

Crystal Violet (*Viola Crystallina*) B.P. syn. Medicinal Gentian Violet is hexamethyl*para*rosanaline hydrochloride, one of the group of dyes derived from triphenylmethane, and contains at least 96 per cent of ($[CH_3]_2N\cdot C_6H_4)_2C:C_6H_4:N(CH_3)_2\cdot Cl$. It occurs as greenish-bronze crystals or powder. It is a deep violet colour in solution. Crystal violet is soluble 1 part in 200 parts of water, 1 in 30 of glycerin and is very soluble in alcohol.

Crystal violet is incompatible with sodium chloride, and with other electrolytes, and with sodium lauryl sulphate.

Fresh stains of crystal violet may be removed from the skin with Aromatic Spirit of Ammonia (Sal Volatile).

Crystal violet is a powerful antiseptic with a selective action against Gram-positive organisms. It is quite ineffective against Gram-negative organisms. Crystal violet is also used as a fungicide. 1–2 per cent solutions of crystal violet in spirit are markedly astringent and have been used with success on soft corns, small warts, macerated plantar callus, etc. It does appear that solution of gentian violet, which is not so pure as crystal violet, is more effective than the latter as an astringent. For direct application to the skin as a fungicidal paint a 1:1,000 solution in water is generally used.

Because it is effective only against certain groups of organisms, crystal violet is frequently combined with other similar drugs which are effective against other groups of pathogenic organisms, the combined drugs having a wider range of antibacterial activity. Care must be taken when applying the dyes to prevent the obliteration of skin lesions, otherwise it may be difficult to observe progress or regression.

Crystal Violet and Brilliant Green Paint (Pigmentum Tinctorum) B.P.C. 1954 contains 0·5 per cent of Crystal Violet and 0·5 per cent of Brilliant Green in Alcohol and Water. This is a non-irritant antiseptic for sterilizing the skin and for the treatment of septic conditions. It is applied as a paint.

Compound Crystal Violet Paint (Pigmentum Violae Crystallinae Compositum) B.P.C. 1954 syn. Triple Dye contains 0·229 per cent of Crystal Violet, 0·229 per cent of Brilliant Green and 0·114 per cent of Proflavine Hemisulphate in water to 100 per cent. This compound paint is effective against a wide range of pathogenic organisms both Gram-positive and Gram-negative and may be employed as an antiseptic paint.

DIBROMOPROPAMIDINE ISETHIONATE

Dibromopropamidine Isethionate (*Dibromopropamidinae Isethionas*) B.P.C. is an aromatic diamidine. It occurs as a white crystalline solid which is soluble 1 part in 2 parts of water and 1 in 60 of alcohol.

Dibromopropamidine isethionate is bactericidal and fungistatic and is active against streptococci and against *Staphylococcus aureus* and also against certain Gram-negative bacteria, notably *Escherichia coli, Proteus vulgaris* and some strains of *Pseudomonas pyocyanea*. It is used in the form of a cream for the treatment of burns, small wounds and abrasions and also of septic conditions. The cream may be used also in the treatment of dermatophytosis. The cream should be applied liberally and covered with a sterile dressing.

A 0·15 per cent cream is particularly effective against penicillin-resistant Staphylococci.

"Brulidine Cream" (May & Baker) is an oil-in-water cream containing 0·15 per cent w/w dibromopropamidine isethionate.

"Johnson's First Aid Cream" (Johnson & Johnson) contains Dibromopropamidine isethionate 0·2 per cent and Lignocaine hydrochloride 0·05 per cent in a water-miscible base.

DICHLOROACETIC ACID

Dichloroacetic Acid $CHCl_2 \cdot COOH$ is a colourless liquid with the characteristic vinegary odour of the chloroacetic acids.

Dichloroacetic acid is caustic and keratolytic and is used in the treatment of warts and of callus.

In the treatment of warts, dichloroacetic acid is used in a mixture named for convenience, *Tri-acid*, which consists of:

Monochloroacetic acid	3 parts
Dichloroacetic acid	2 parts
Trichloroacetic acid	1 part

It is used in the same way as monochloroacetic acid, but results in a somewhat cheesy coagulum instead of the slough often produced by monochloroacetic acid when used alone. The return period is from 5–14 days and is generally 7 days. Dichloroacetic acid may also be used with Toughened Silver Nitrate in the treatment of large shallow moist growths. The technique of application is the same as for the application of trichloroacetic acid with Toughened Silver Nitrate.

In the treatment of callus the method used is as follows:

1. Remove as much as possible of the callus with the knife.

2. Paint round the callus with Collodion of Ichthammol or with collodion which has been coloured with a dye.

3. Paint the callus with dichloroacetic acid and allow it to dry. (The dichloroacetic acid may fume in contact with the air.)

4. Pad and strap in the usual way, or cover the callus with adhesive stockinette. The return period is 14 days.

When the patient returns, a dirty grey coagulum will be seen, the edges of which will have curled up leaving healthy tissue underneath. In many cases the coagulum may be peeled off with forceps. If this treatment is repeated over a number of visits, the callus will be considerably reduced in size and may be entirely eliminated. This technique is indicated in cases of heavy plantar callus, including those associated with hyperidrosis.

DOMIPHEN BROMIDE

Domiphen Bromide (*Domiphenis Bromidum*) B.P. Trade name: "Bradosol" (Ciba) occurs as colourless or faintly yellow flakes which are readily soluble in water and alcohol.

Domiphen Bromide is a quaternary ammonium compound and is a cationic detergent. Its action is inhibited by soaps and the anionic detergents. It should be stored away from the light. It is incompatible with proflavine and potassium hydroxide.

Domiphen Bromide may be used as a 0·5 per cent solution in 70 per cent isopropyl alcohol as a pre-operative antiseptic and a 0·05 aqueous solution as a wound antiseptic or for instrument storage (with sodium nitrite added). Domiphen Bromide has antifungal activity and may be used in the treatment of skin infections.

"ENTONOX"

"Entonox" (British Oxygen) is a mixture of equal volumes of Nitrous Oxide and Oxygen. Administered by inhalation it produces analgesia and relieves anxiety. It is generally used "on demand"— the patients operating the apparatus for themselves. Generally there are no side effects and an adequate degree of analgesia can be attained after a few deep inhalations. "Entonox" mixture must not be allowed to drop below a temperature of 0° C.

ETHER

Solvent Ether (*Aether Solvens*) B.P. is di-ethyl ether:

$$C_2H_5-O-C_2H_5$$

obtained by the distillation of a mixture of sulphuric acid and ethyl alcohol, the distillate being re-distilled to purify it. Solvent ether has a specific gravity of 0·72 and a flash point of − 29° C.

Technical Ether or Methylated Ether is prepared from Industrial Methylated Spirit instead of ethyl alcohol and is subsequently denatured by the addition of wood naphtha (cf. Methylated Spirit).

Ether should be stored in dark, well-stoppered bottles in a cool place.

Ether is a light liquid which is very volatile and highly inflammable.

It gives off a vapour which is two-and-a-half times as heavy as air and which is liable to "creep" along the floor. Since the vapour forms an explosive mixture with oxygen it is extremely dangerous to leave a bottle of ether unstoppered if there is any sort of open fire or electrical apparatus in the room. The vapour from discarded swabs will tend to remain in the dirty dressing bin, but is nevertheless a potential source of danger.

Solvent ether or technical ether is used in chiropody to dissolve grease and rubber adhesive from the skin. Its pungent odour is a disadvantage but it is a satisfactory adhesive solvent and will remove plaster marks from the skin. It is particularly effective when the rubber adhesive mass is old and has dried out. Its very efficiency as a solvent is sometimes a disadvantage especially if the plaster mass is fresh. Because it is a good solvent the ether rapidly becomes saturated with the rubber adhesive and because it is also very volatile it evaporates rapidly, leaving a thin film of rubber adhesive on the skin, which feels sticky.

It must be remembered at all times that ether is potentially a dangerous explosive.

ETHYL ACETATE

Ethyl Acetate (*Aethylis Acetas*) B.P. App. Ia. syn. Acetic Ether has the formula $CH_3 \cdot COO \cdot C_2H_5$ and is a transparent liquid with a fragrant odour. Ethyl Acetate boils in the range of 75–78° C. It should be stored in a cool place.

Ethyl Acetate is used in Chiropody as a solvent for the removal of rubber plaster mass from the skin prior to operating and is the solvent of choice since it has neither the toxic manifestations of Carbon Tetrachloride nor the explosive potential of Ether.

It is also used in the manufacture of appliances as a solvent for "Samcoforma" and as a general-purpose solvent.

ETHYL ALCOHOL (see Alcohol)

ETHYL CHLORIDE

Ethyl Chloride (*Aethylis Chloridum*) B.P. contains not less than 99·5 per cent w/w of C_2H_5Cl. Ethyl chloride is gaseous at ordinary temperatures but when slightly compressed it is a colourless, mobile liquid. It is very volatile and is highly inflammable. Ethyl chloride is usually stored in a small glass cylinder known as an anestile. It should be stored in a cool place away from the light.

Ethyl chloride is a local anaesthetic. As the liquid is released from pressure, the jet from the anestile is played upon the area to be anaesthetized. The rapid evaporation of the liquid freezes the area which becomes numb: there is, however, considerable pain when the part thaws.

Ethyl chloride is sometimes used to assist in the treatment of onychocryptosis during the removal of the splinter, but when the ethyl chloride has frozen the tissues it becomes a question of finding a comparatively soft nail splinter imbedded in hard surroundings, instead of a hard nail splinter in soft surroundings. The whole area will also have been blanched a uniform white colour. Ethyl chloride is therefore not a very practical aid to chiropodial treatment.

EUCALYPTUS OIL (see Oils, Essential)

EUFLAVINE (see Amino-acridines)

FATS, ANIMAL

Wool Fat (*Adeps Lanae*) B.P. syn. Anhydrous Lanolin is the purified, anhydrous, fat-like substance obtained from the wool of the sheep, *Ovis aries*. It is a pale yellow tenacious substance with a faint characteristic odour. It melts at 36–42° C. Wool fat is insoluble in water, sparingly soluble in alcohol but is readily soluble in ether and acetone.

Hydrous Wool Fat (*Adeps Lanae Hydrosus*) B.P. syn. Lanolin consists of Wool Fat 70 per cent with water 30 per cent.

Simple Ointment (*Unguentum Simplex*) B.P. contains 5 per cent of Wool Fat, 5 per cent of Hard Paraffin, 5 per cent of Cetostearyl Alcohol and 85 per cent of White or Yellow Soft Paraffin.

Hydrous Wool Fat Ointment (*Unguentum Adipis Lanae Hydrosi*) B.P.C. syn. Lanolin Ointment contains equal parts of Hydrous Wool Fat and Yellow Soft Paraffin.

Wool fat closely resembles the sebaceous secretion of the human skin. Contrary to general belief it is not itself easily absorbed, but mixed with vegetable oils, or "fats" such as white or yellow soft paraffin, it gives an emollient cream which penetrates the hair follicles and assists the absorption of medicaments. Since it can absorb about 30 per cent of water, wool fat is used to prepare water-in-oil emulsions.

Hydrous wool fat is frequently used as an ointment base, especially for medicaments in aqueous solution. Soft or liquid paraffin is generally added to reduce the stickiness and to make a smooth penetrating ointment. Hydrous wool fat is a favourite emollient amongst chiropodists and Lanolin, or Lanolin Ointment, is frequently recommended for home use by those who have dry skins.

Wool Alcohols (*Alcoholia Lanae*) B.P. is a crude mixture of steroid and triterpene alcohols obtained by treating wool fat with alkalies and separating the fractions containing cholesterol and other alcohols. It contains not less than 28 per cent of cholesterol. It is a golden-brown solid melting at not lower than 58° C. It is insoluble in water, partly soluble in alcohol and readily soluble in ether.

Incorporated in water-in-oil emulsions, wool alcohols increase the quantity of water which may be incorporated in the emulsion, and improves the texture, stability and emollient properties of the emulsion.

Wool Alcohols Ointment (*Unguentum Alcoholium Lanae*) B.P. contains 6 per cent of Wool Alcohols, 24 per cent of Hard Paraffin, 10 per cent of Soft Paraffin and 60 per cent of Liquid Paraffin.

Oily Cream, syn. *Hydrous Ointment* B.P. contains 50 per cent of Wool Alcohols Ointment and 50 per cent of water.

"Eucerin Anhydrous" (Smith & Nephew) is a proprietary preparation corresponding to Wool Alcohols Ointment. "Eucerin Hydrous" corresponds to Oily Cream.

"Nivea Creme" is a similar but lighter preparation.

FERRIC SALTS (see Iron)

FORMALDEHYDE

Formaldehyde ($H \cdot CHO$) is a gas prepared by the oxidation of methyl alcohol with atmospheric oxygen using copper as a catalyst. Some methyl alcohol is left in the product in order to prevent polymerization.

Formaldehyde Solution (*Liquor Formaldehydi*) B.P. This solution is known in Great Britain and Northern Ireland as Formalin (in other parts of the world "Formalin" is a Trade Mark) and is a saturated solution of the gas in water and contains 37–41 per cent of $H \cdot CHO$. "1 per cent solution of formalin" and "1 per cent of formaldehyde" both indicate 1 per cent of this solution.

Formaldehyde Solution is a colourless liquid with a pungent odour. A white deposit may form in the liquid on storage.

Formalin is astringent, disinfectant and fungicidal. It has the effect of hardening the skin and reducing the apparent secretion of sweat. (See chapter on Hyperidrosis.)

Formaldehyde Solution may be used:

1. As an astringent and hardening foot-bath for hyperidrosis or

bromidrosis in a strength of 1:200–1:800. (One tablespoonful to a gallon of water gives a 1:320 solution.) The temperature of the water should be cool in order to minimize the vaporization of the formalin which may cause irritation of the eyes, nose and throat. The foot-bath should be followed by a rinse with plain water. This treatment was very effective in hardening the feet of recruits in the Army.

2. A 10 per cent solution of formaldehyde may be used *as a paint* in severe cases of hyperidrosis and bromidrosis. This is a very effective treatment but it should not be used more than once a week and may well be used at longer intervals.

3. A 10 per cent suspension of formaldehyde in collodion may be used to treat warts. A 3–5 per cent solution in water may also be used, the warts being soaked daily in the solution by the patient at home. The skin surrounding the warts should be protected with a smear of petroleum jelly. A saucer is a suitable vessel for containing the solution. The patient should report to the surgery once a week for the removal of the hardened tissue. This method is very effective in the treatment of certain mosaic warts. In some cases it is more convenient to apply a stronger solution of formaldehyde in the surgery. This avoids the danger of the solution being applied to the normal skin. For a 40 per cent solution applied in the surgery the return period is 7 days.

4. Formalin is now available 1·5 per cent in a water-miscible gel ("Veracur," Typharm, Blanford Forum, Dorset). The gel may be applied daily to warts and covered with adhesive dressing.

5. Formaldehyde Solution may be employed as a fumigant for shoes. A tin lid containing Formaldehyde Solution is placed in the shoes to be fumigated, and the shoes are wrapped in newspaper and left for 24 hours. This method may be employed when a patient has a severe fungal infection and serves to prevent reinfection from the shoes.

6. Formaldehyde Solution may be employed in the cold sterilization of instruments.

7. Formaldehyde vapour is the active agent in "Bacterol" sterilizers.

Paraformaldehyde (*Paraformaldehydum*) B.P.C. is the solid polymeride of formaldehyde which is sometimes used to produce formalin vapour for the purpose of sterilizing footwear.

"Formagene Tablets" (Evans Medical Supplies) are disinfectant tablets which liberate Formalin in the form of a vapour.

Acetaldehyde, $CH_3 \cdot CHO$, is more effective than formaldehyde as a fumigant for shoes and has the advantage that its vapour is less irritant than that of formaldehyde. Swabs of cotton wool saturated with acetaldehyde may be placed in the shoes which are then wrapped in newspaper as in (5) above.

GLUTARALDEHYDE

Glutaraldehyde, Glutaric Dialdehyde, Prop: Cidex $CHO \cdot (CH_2)_3 \cdot CHO$ is a liquid, soluble in water and alchohol. It is less irritant to the skin than Formaldehyde but it may cause sensitization.

Glutaraldehyde is a disinfectant which is rapidly effective against vegetative forms of Gram positive and Gram negative bacteria. It is also Fungicidal. It may be used for instrument sterilization as a 2 per cent solution. Disinfection takes place in 15–20 minutes but exposure for 3 hours is required for complete sterilization. It is rapidly effective against serum hepatitis type B antigen and may be used as "extra" sterilization procedure (page 75). All instruments used on a patient are kept isolated in a separate instrument tray or better on a clean paper towel which can be discarded. When operating has been completed the used instruments should be washed under running water and immersed for at least 10 minutes in 2 per cent glutaraldehyde solution and should be washed again before being returned to the instrument tray which should contain an antiseptic such as Chlorhexidine (page 178) or "Savlon" (page 162).

"Cidex" (Ethicon) is a 2 per cent Solution of Glutaraldehyde. An activating powder is added before use which makes a buffered alkaline solution which is stable for 14 days. The activator also acts as a rust-inhibitor.

Glutaraldehyde solutions of 5 or 10 per cent have been used in the treatment of hyperidosis. A 10 per cent solution has been used in the treatment of Onychomycosis. Superficial infections may be cured in 4–6 weeks but full thickness infections require treatment for 4–6 months.

HALOGENATED PHENOLS

Chlorocresol (*Chlorocresol*) B.P. is 4-chloro-3-methylphenol and occurs as colourless crystals with a characteristic phenolic odour. It is soluble 1 part in 260 parts of water and is soluble in alcohol and ether.

Chlorocresol is a powerful germicide of low toxicity. It is used as a preservative in many Creams.

Chloroxylenol (*Chloroxylenol*) B.P. is 4-chloro-3,5-xylenol. Chloroxylenol occurs as white or creamy-white crystals which are soluble 1 part in 6,000 parts of water, and soluble in alcohol, ether, terpenes, fixed oils, and in solutions of alkaline hydroxides.

It is chiefly used as:

Chloroxylenol Solution (*Liquor Chloroxylenolis*) B.P.C. syn. Roxenol (for trade names see below) contains Chloroxylenol 5 per cent, Terpineol 10 per cent, (95 per cent) Alcohol 20 per cent, Castor Oil 6·3 per cent, Potassium Hydroxide 1·36 per cent, and Oleic Acid 0·15 per cent.

Roxenol is an amber coloured liquid with the clinging odour of terpineol. With nineteen times its own volume of water it forms a stable white emulsion.

Chloroxylenol is a powerful and non-irritant bactericide of low toxicity. It exerts a selective action against streptococci, is less effective against staphylococci and it is almost inactive against certain of the Gram-negative organisms such as *Pseudomonas pyocyanea*. It is therefore a less reliable antiseptic than Lysol but is very much less caustic and less irritant to the skin and is, therefore, more popular. It can be used in effective strength on the skin without causing damage, whereas Lysol cannot.

Chloroxylenol Solution may be used undiluted for instrument sterilization and as a 2 per cent solution in water for the storage of instruments in the instrument tray, without damaging the instruments, provided that it is not contaminated with caustic chemicals. Chloroxylenol Solution may be used as a foot-bath 120 ml. (4 oz.) to 5 litres (1 gallon) of water, for septic conditions or as a deodorant in cases of bromidrosis and hyperidrosis. Chloroxylenol Solution is contra-indicated as a wet dressing for wounds and abrasions. The pure solution, or a cream containing chloroxylenol such as is prepared for obstetric use, may be rubbed into the operator's hands prior to handling a septic case and will afford a fair measure of protection.

Chloroxylenol is the active principle in a number of non-irritant, non-toxic germicides by various makers including:

"Antiseptol" (Malam Laboratories), "Asterit" (Laporte Chemicals), "C.M.X. Antiseptic" (Wyleys), "Dettol" (Reckitt & Sons), "G.P. Germicide" (Cuxson, Gerrard), "Gardal" (Pigot & Smith), "Gomaxide" (Gomax Ltd.), "Hewsol" (Astra-Hewlett), "Hycolin" (William Pearson Ltd.), "Ibcol Extra" (Jeyes), "Jeypine" (Jeyes), "Monsol Disinfectant" (Leonard Smith), "Neo-Monsol Germicide" (Leonard Smith), "O-Syl" (Lehn & Fink), "Prinsyl" (Printar), "Pynol" (Cooper, McDougall & Robertson), "Supersan" (Boots), "Zal" (Izal Ltd.), "Zant" (Evans Medical).

"Dettol Obstetric Cream" (Reckitt & Sons) is a non-greasy preparation containing 1·4 per cent Chloroxylenol and 1·8 per cent

Terpineol. "Dettol Ointment" contains Chloroxylenol 3 per cent, Salicylic Acid 0·2 per cent and Menthol 0·2 per cent.

"Instrument Dettol" contains Chloroxylenol 6 per cent, Terpineol 12·5 per cent. It forms a clear solution with either soft or distilled water.

"Hycolin" (William Pearson Ltd.) contains a mixture of halogenated phenols including chlorocresol and chloroxylenol.

"Hycolin Antibacterial Cream" for use as an antiseptic hand cream contains 2·5 per cent of "Hycolin" and 1 per cent of Hexachlorophane. "Hycolin Antibacterial Liquid Hand Soap" contains "Hycolin" 5 per cent and Hexachlorophane 2 per cent.

Chlorhexidine Gluconate Solution B.P. is a 20 per cent aqueous solution of Chlorhexidine Gluconate 1,6-di(N-p-chlorophenyl-diguanido) hexane digluconate. It is an almost colourless or straw-coloured liquid with a bitter taste. It is miscible with water and alcohol.

Chlorhexidine Acetate B.P.C. and **Chlorhexidine Hydrochloride** B.P. are of similar chemical composition but are the acetate and hydrochloride respectively. They are powders.

Chlorhexidine is incompatible with soaps and anionic detergents.

Chlorhexidine solutions are inactivated by cork, and cork closures should not be used for containers of chlorhexidine solution.

Chlorhexidine is a useful topical antiseptic and is active against a wide range of Gram-positive and Gram-negative bacteria. It has a wide range of uses as a general antiseptic and may also be used for a pre- and post-operative application, for instrument sterilization and storage. For the treatment of wounds solutions containing 0·02 to 0·1 per cent are used. For pre- and post-operative application to the skin a 0·5 solution in alcohol or a 0·5 per cent aqueous solution may be used. In the instrument tray a 0·1 per cent aqueous solution with added sodium nitrite may be used. For the rapid (1–2 minutes) sterilization of instruments a 0·5 per cent solution in 70 per cent alcohol is recommended.

Chlorhexidine hydrochloride should be used in preference to the gluconate where a prolonged action is required.

Chlorhexidine Cream (*Cremor Chlorhexidinae*) B.P.C. contains 0·1 per cent of Chlorhexidine Gluconate in a cream basis.

Chlorhexidine Dusting-powder B.P.C. contains 0·5 per cent of Chlorhexidine Hydrochloride in Absorbable Dusting-powder.

"Hibitane" (I.C.I.) is chlorhexidine available as the acetate or hydrochloride or as a 20 per cent solution of the gluconate.

"Hibitane Concentrate" (I.C.I.) contains 5 per cent of Chlorhexidine Gluconate with a surface active agent. Hibitane is also available as "Hibitane Antiseptic Cream" 1 per cent in a water miscible basis and as "Hibitane Industrial Cream" 1 per cent as a hand cream.

"Hibitane Aerosol" gives a 1 per cent solution of Hibitane in isopropyl alcohol for skin disinfection.

Hexachlorophane B.P. syn. Hexachlorophene is 2, 2'-methylenebis (3, 4, 6-trichlorophenol). It is a white or pale buff crystalline powder which is insoluble in water but is soluble 1 in 3·5 of alcohol.

Hexachlorophane is active against a wide variety of organisms and is more active against Gram-positive than Gram-negative organisms. Its chief advantage is that it is compatible with, and retains its activity in the presence of, soap. It is chiefly used as an antiseptic in soaps and creams in strength of from 1–3 per cent. Skin sensitization has been known to occur following the repeated use of hexachlorophane but its advantages greatly outweigh the disadvantages.

Hexachlorophane Dusting-powder B.P.C. contains 0·3 per cent Hexachlorophane, 3 per cent Zinc Oxide in a basis of Absorbable Dusting Powder.

Hexachlorophane is an ingredient of:

"Cidal Soap" (Bibby) 2 per cent, "Disfex" (Pigot & Smith) 3 per cent, "Gramophen Surgical Soap" (Ethicon) 2 per cent, "Hexabalm" (Christie, George) 0·5 per cent cream, "pHisoHex" Bayer Products) 3 per cent cream, "Sebbix Soap" (Fisons Pharmaceuticals) 2 per cent, "Steriloderm" (Willows Francis) 0·01 per cent gel, "Ster-Zac Antibacterial Soap" (Hough) 2 per cent, also as liquid soap 3 per cent. "Zalpon Antibacterial Washing Cream" (Izal Ltd.) 2·5 per cent, and "Zeasorb Powder" (Stiefel) 0·5 per cent, antiseptic dusting-powder.

HAMAMELIS

Hamamelis Extract, Liquid (Extractum Hamamelidis Siccum) B.P.C. is prepared from Powdered Hamamelis obtained from the dried leaves of *Hamamelis virginiana*.

Hamamelis Water (Aqua Hamamelidis) B.P.C. is a solution prepared from the fresh leaves and twigs of the *Hamamelis virginiana*. The active principles are tannin and hamamelis.

Hamamelis Water (Witch Hazel) is soothing, astringent and haemostatic. It is a clear, odourless liquid with a characteristic odour. It has a direct effect on the blood vessels, acting as a vasoconstrictor.

Witch Hazel may be used as a compress to reduce acute inflammation in cases of acute bursitis, chilblains, bruising and lacerations. It may also be used as a compress to alleviate the inflammation set up by the acids, silver nitrate, etc. It may be used to reduce the inflammation in plaster rash or iodine rash.

Hamamelis Ointment (*Unguentum Hamamelidis*) B.P.C. contains 10 per cent of Liquid extract of Hamamelis, 50 per cent of Wool Fat and 40 per cent of Yellow Soft Paraffin. It is a soothing ointment.

"Hazeldine Brand Witchazel Cream" (Burroughs Wellcome) is an emollient cream containing Witch Hazel in a base closely resembling the natural oily secretion of the skin.

HEXACHLOROPHANE (see Halogenated Phenols)

HYDRARGAPHEN (see Mercury)

HYDROGEN PEROXIDE (SOLUTION)

Hydrogen Peroxide Solution (*Liquor Hydrogenii Peroxidi*) B.P. is an aqueous solution of Hydrogen Peroxide H_2O_2, containing from 5–7 per cent w/v of H_2O_2. One ml. of this solution yields about 20 ml. of oxygen and it is known as the "20 Volume" solution. Hydrogen peroxide solution is comparatively stable when it is slightly acid but decomposes rapidly when it is alkaline or when it is in contact with oxidizable materials.

Hydrogen peroxide solution is incompatible with most organic substances and with alkalies, iodides, potassium permanganate and with other oxidizable materials. Hydrogen peroxide solution is best used by itself, although it may be followed by practically any of the common wound antiseptics.

Hydrogen peroxide solutions are also obtainable in 10-, 12-, 30- and 100-volume strengths.

Hydrogen Peroxide Solution exerts a direct antiseptic action on bacteria, especially anaerobic bacteria which are particularly sensitive to it. Aerobic bacteria secrete an enzyme, catalase, which rapidly breaks down hydrogen peroxide to oxygen and water. This serves as a useful test for the differential diagnosis of septic and non-septic exudates. A few drops of hydrogen peroxide solution applied to a non-septic exudate will bubble quietly, but if applied to a septic exudate violent effervescence will take place.

Hydrogen Peroxide Solution may be employed as a mechanical cleansing agent for septic cavities, fissures and nail sulci. The effervescence may help to loosen pus and debris. For this purpose it is generally used diluted with an equal volume of distilled water. Applied to the nail groove, Hydrogen Peroxide Solution softens the accumulated debris and greatly facilitates the clearing of the groove with an excavator. The softening action of the hydrogen peroxide is enhanced if the debris is loosened slightly before the solution is applied.

The use of hydrogen peroxide is not to be recommended on large areas of ulceration especially those where healing is impaired. It is suggested that it may be toxic when absorbed.

Hydrogen Peroxide Solution has been used as a styptic. Applied with digital pressure, it will control most of the capillary haemorrhages encountered in chiropody. Any of the common wound antiseptics may be used as an after-dressing.

Hydrogen peroxide solutions should be stored in dark, glass-stoppered bottles in a cool place. Tightly stoppered bottles of the solution have been known to explode and therefore the stoppers of containers of hydrogen peroxide should always be loosened, so that if rapid decomposition of the solution should take place the stopper will be forced out.

"Genoxide" (Laporte Chemicals) is a proprietary brand of Hydrogen Peroxide Solution B.P.

ICHTHAMMOL

Ichthammol (*Ichthammol*) B.P. syn. Ammonium Ichthosulphonate, Ichthyol, Subitine is a viscous, almost black substance, with a disagreeable odour and consists chiefly of the ammonium salts of the sulphonic acids of an oil prepared from a bituminous schist consisting of the remains of marine animals, with ammonium sulphate and water.

Ichthammol is soluble in water, partly soluble in 90 per cent alcohol and is miscible with glycerin.

Ichthammol is a mild antiseptic and is said to stimulate healing and healthy granulation. It tends to liquify pus.

Ichthammol Glycerin (*Glycerinum Ichthammolis*) B.P.C. contains 10 per cent of Ichthammol in 90 per cent Glycerin.

Ichthammol Ointment (*Unguentum Ichthammolis*) B.P.C. contains 10 per cent of Ichthammol in 45 per cent of Wool Fat and 45 per cent of Yellow Soft Paraffin.

Zinc and Ichthammol Cream (*Cremor Zinci et Ichthammolis*) B.P.C. contains 5 per cent of Ichthammol, 3 per cent Cetostearyl Alcohol, 10 per cent of Wool Fat in Zinc Cream to 100 per cent.

A preparation of Ichthammol 12·5 per cent in Simple Collodion to 100 per cent is also used, particularly when maceration and sogginess are to be avoided, when a paint is required or when a cotton dressing is contra-indicated.

Ichthammol obstinately retains its place in chiropody practice although it is gradually being replaced by more effective modern drugs. It is not indicated for the treatment of most ulcers. The use of Ichthammol is distinctly old-fashioned but it has been used widely for many years.

On the ulcers left after the breakdown of warts by acids, Ichthammol in Collodion may be used. Chilblains in general and broken chilblains in particular may be painted with Ichthammol in Collodion or may be dressed with Glycerin of Ichthammol or Ichthammol Ointment. Deep fissures, whether moist or dry, may be painted with Ichthammol in Collodion.

The breakdown which is sometimes found when reducing a hypertrophied nail responds well when treated with Ichthammol in Collodion. A dressing of cotton wool, soaked in Ichthammol in Collodion, is placed over the nail and allowed to dry in position. This forms an effective occlusive dressing and healing takes place uninterrupted underneath the dressing.

IODINE

Iodine (*Iodum*) B.P. occurs as heavy bluish-black rhombic crystals or plates, having a metallic lustre and containing not less than 99·5 per cent of Iodine.

Iodine is slightly soluble in water: soluble one part in twelve parts of alcohol, and one in four of ether, and is readily soluble in aqueous solutions of the iodides.

Iodine is incompatible with alkalies, alkaloids, starch, the soluble salts of lead, mercury, and silver, with phenol and with sodium thiosulphate. Iodine forms a disagreeable pungent compound with acetone.

Some patients, notably those with very fair skins, have an idiosyncrasy to Iodine which gives rise to an erythematous rash. Iodine rash may be treated with Starch Glycerin B.P.C. 1963 or with a compress of a 1:200 aqueous solution of sodium thiosulphate. Iodine burns may be treated in a similar way. Solutions of iodine may increase in strength during storage due to the corrosion of the cork of the container and subsequent evaporation of the solution. Iodine and solutions of iodine must always be stored in glass-stoppered bottles, or in glass or earthenware containers with well-waxed bungs.

Iodine in solution is germicidal on the intact skin only, losing its germicidal power in the presence of organic material. Solutions of iodine are also fungicidal and rubefacient. Ointments containing iodine are rubefacient and may be emollient by virtue of their bases. Iodine Oil is a useful rubefacient.

Iodine Solution, Aqueous (*Liquor Iodi Aequosus*) B.P. syn. Lugol's

Solution contains 5 per cent of Iodine, 10 per cent of Potassium Iodide in water to 100 per cent.

Strong Iodine Solution (Liquor Iodi Fortis) B.P. 1958 contains 10 per cent of Iodine, 6 per cent of Potassium Iodide in 10 per cent of water and (90 per cent) Alcohol to 100 per cent.

Strong Iodine Solution may be used as a rubefacient paint for chronic or subacute bursitis. For chilblains it may be applied as a paint diluted with an equal volume of Compound Benzoin Tincture, or may be painted on to the lesions and followed with a coat of Compound Benzoin Tincture. As a fungicide, Strong Iodine Solution is particularly useful in cases of onychomycosis, but it may also be applied to other forms of mycotic infection either alone or with Compound Benzoin Tincture.

Weak Iodine Solution (Liquor Iodi Mitis) B.P. contains 2·5 per cent of Iodine, 2·5 per cent of Potassium Iodide in water 2·5 per cent and Alcohol (90 per cent) to 100 per cent.

Weak Iodine Solution may be used as a pre- or post-operative antiseptic paint on the unbroken skin. When applied to the skin it exerts a mild, lasting irritation and produces some subcutaneous congestion. Weak Iodine Solution may be used as a daily paint for chilblains either alone or mixed with an equal volume of Compound Benzoin Tincture. Weak Iodine Solution is sometimes used to promote the absorption of fluid in chronic or subacute bursitis but the Strong Solution is more frequently used for this purpose.

Iodine Ointment, Non-staining (Unguentum Iodi Denigrescens) B.P.C. contains 5 per cent of Iodine in 15 per cent of Arachis Oil and Yellow Soft Paraffin to 100 per cent.

Iodine Ointment, Non-staining, with Methyl Salicylate (Unguentum Iodi Denigrescens cum Methylis Salicylate) B.P.C. contains 5 per cent of Methyl Salicylate with Non-staining Ointment of Iodine to 100 per cent.

Non-staining Iodine Ointment is a bland ointment which may be used repeatedly and which may be applied to broken surfaces. When the Non-staining Iodine Ointment is combined with Methyl Salicylate it has an additional rubefacient and analgesic action but it may not then be applied to broken surfaces. Inunction of Iodine Ointment is helped by the action of heat. These ointments are indicated in cases of chronic congestion, chilblains and bursitis and they have an emollient action by virtue of their base. They are also useful ointments to employ in buffer pads although it is not advisable to use the ointment containing Methyl Salicylate for this purpose because it may produce maceration.

"Iodex" (Smith Kline & French) is a stainless Iodine Ointment containing 4 per cent of Iodine and it may also be obtained combined with 5 per cent of Methyl Salicylate.

Iodobenz is a paint which has proved beneficial in the stages of chilblains where a rubefacient is required.

The preparation may be made from the following constituents:

Resublimed Iodine . . .	2·5 grammes
Menthol B.P.	1·0 gramme
Isopropyl Alcohol	23 ml.
Flexible Collodion B.P. . . .	50 ml.
Compound Benzoin Tincture to . .	100 ml.

Iodochlorhydroxyquinoline syn. Clioquinol is a stable powder containing 41 per cent of Iodine.

"Vioform" (Ciba) is a 3 per cent cream of clioquinol useful as a wound antiseptic. "Vioform" is apt to stain clothing and precautions should be taken to prevent this happening.

Povidone-Iodine (U.S.N.F.) contains 9–12 per cent of available iodine in a complex with Polyvidone which gives the advantages of iodine without producing the allergic manifestations.

"Betadine" (Berk Pharmaceuticals) is Povidone-Iodine, available as an antiseptic solution or ointment containing 1 per cent of available iodine or as an aerosol spray with 0·75 per cent of available iodine.

Povidone-Iodine is an example of an "iodophore". Iodophores are usually complexes of iodine with certain surface active agents. They are frequently used for general disinfectant purposes in industry, particularly in the food and dairy industries. They may also be used for the disinfection of swimming pools, shower baths etc.

IRON

Solutions of ferric chloride are incompatible with tannin, the iodides, alkalies, alkaline carbonates, salicylates (including T.C.P.), and silver salts.

Ferric Chloride Solution (Liquor Ferri Perchloridi) B.P.C. contains from 13·9 to 16·1 per cent of Ferric Chloride and is prepared by dilution of the strong Solution 1 part to 3 parts water.

Ferric Chloride Solution may be used as a styptic, or it may be applied daily for one week to a relaxed nail sulcus in order to harden the tissues. It may be applied twice daily to hypergranulation tissue associated with onychocryptosis.

Ferric Chloride Solution, Strong (Liquor Ferri Perchloridi Fortis) B.P.C. is prepared by the interaction of iron with hydrochloric and nitric acids and contains about 60 per cent of Ferric Chloride.

Ferric Chloride Solution, Strong is a powerful astringent and may be applied to a relaxed nail sulcus, to hypergranulation tissue or to vascular corns. In each of these instances the Ferric Chloride Solution, Strong, should be painted on in the surgery not more than twice a week.

Solutions of Ferric Chloride are contra-indicated in weeping skin conditions.

ISOPROPYL ALCOHOL (see Alcohols)

KAOLIN

Heavy Kaolin (*Kaolinum Ponderosum*) B.P. syn. China Clay is a native, white hydrated aluminium silicate. It is a soft white powder, insoluble in all ordinary solvents and in the mineral acids.

Light Kaolin (*Kaolinum Leve*) B.P. has particles of a smaller size than those of Heavy Kaolin.

Powdered light kaolin is employed for its absorbent and anti-pruritic qualities, in dusting-powders. Kaolin must be carefully sterilized before it is dispensed as a powder because it may be contaminated with the anaerobic bacteria *Clostridium welchii*, *Cl. tetani*, etc. It is always wiser not to use dusting-powders containing kaolin on abraded surfaces.

Kaolin may be used as a paste made with water, in cases of chilblains and heavy plantar callus. The paste is applied spread on lint.

Kaolin Poultice (*Cataplasma Kaolini*) B.P. contains 52·7 per cent of Heavy Kaolin with Boric Acid 4·5 per cent, Methyl Salicylate 0·2 per cent, Peppermint Oil 0·05 per cent, Thymol 0·05 per cent and Glycerin to 100 per cent.

There are many products closely resembling Kaolin Poultice, perhaps the best known being "Antiphlogistine" (Denver Chemical Co.).

Kaolin Poultice is employed as a vehicle for the application of moist heat to local inflammation. Applied to an open septic wound Kaolin Poultice also absorbs pus and other discharges. The poultice is best applied at a temperature of about 50° C. Kaolin Poultice having raised the temperature of the tissues helps to maintain the raised temperature by acting as an insulator and preventing loss of heat by radiation. A single thickness of gauze is often applied between the poultice and the wound in order to facilitate the removal of the poultice. Kaolin Poultice is generally left on for 24 hours, unless it can be renewed by the patient at home, when it may be renewed every four hours. The patient should be warned not to apply the poultice at too high a temperature. Kaolin Poultice is often applied to bring underlying sepsis to a head: it may macerate the skin and allow the pus to break through the epidermis and so establish drainage.

Fuller's Earth is a grey or brown native aluminium silicate containing iron, magnesium and calcium as impurities. It is used in dusting-powders.

LACTIC ACID

Lactic Acid (*Acidum Lacticum*) B.P. is a colourless syrupy liquid with a sour taste, containing not less than the equivalent of 87·5 per cent w/w of $CH_3 \cdot CHOH \cdot COOH$. It will mix with water, alcohol and glycerin.

Lactic acid is keratolytic on thickened epidermis and an ointment containing 20–30 per cent of lactic acid may be used in the treatment of corns and warts. It is not widely used in chiropody but there is one important formula:

Lactic acid . . 25 per cent⎫
Salicylic acid . 25 per cent⎭ in a suitable ointment base.

This is a useful caustic for warts, and in particular for those affecting young children. It may be applied in a routine ointment wart dressing (page 109). The foot must be kept out of water during treatment. The return period is 7–14 days.

LEAD

Lead Subacetate Solution, Strong (*Liquor Plumbi Subacetatis Fortis*) B.P.C. contains not less than 19 per cent and not more than 21·5 per cent of Lead. It is prepared from Lead Acetate, Lead Monoxide and Distilled Water.

Lead Subacetate Solution, Dilute (*Liquor Plumbi Subacetatis Dilutis*) B.P.C. contains 1·25 per cent of strong solution of Lead Subacetate diluted to 100 per cent with Distilled Water. It should be freshly prepared.

Lead Subacetate Solution, Dilute, is indicated as a superficial astringent and soothing lotion in all types of inflammation in which the skin is unbroken and the inflammation is not caused by pyogenic bacteria. The lotion relieves congestion. It has a superficial action, because it precipitates both the tissue proteins and also the tissue chlorides, which form an insoluble barrier restricting penetration.

Lead Lotion (*Lotio Plumbi*) B.P.C. is Lead Subacetate Solution, Strong 2·5 per cent in distilled water to 100 per cent. It may be used in lieu of Lead Subacetate Solution, Dilute w ʌen a stronger action is required.

Lead Lotion, Evaporating (*Lotio Plumbi Evaporans*) B.P.C. contains Lead Subacetate Solution, Strong 2·5 per cent in Alcohol (90 per cent) 12·5 per cent and water to 100 per cent.

Lead Plaster Mass (*Emplastrum Plumbi in Massa*) B.P.C. 1954 syn. Diachylon is prepared by boiling together Lead Monoxide and Arachis Oil or Olive Oil. It contains 31–34 per cent of Lead Monoxide. It is sometimes used as a stiff ointment base for salicylic acid.

Lead with Colophony Plaster Mass (*Emplastrum Plumbi cum Colophonio in Massa*) B.P.C. 1954 contains 10 per cent Colophony, 5 per cent of Hard Soap with 85 per cent of Plaster Mass of Lead.

Lead with Soap Plaster Mass (*Emplastrum Plumbi cum Sapone in Massa*) B.P.C. 1954 syn. Saponis contains 2·5 per cent of Colophony, 14 per cent of Hard Soap with 83·5 per cent of Plaster Mass of Lead.

LIGNOCAINE AND RELATED LOCAL ANAESTHETICS

Lignocaine Hydrochloride (*Lignocaini Hydrochloridum*) B.P. is a white powder, which is very soluble in water and alcohol.

Lignocaine is widely used as a local anaesthetic both by injection or applied topically. The general observation that it is difficult to bring the local anaesthetic into contact with nerve endings by topical application in chiropody practice holds true of the use of local anaesthetics generally (see page 15). Lignocaine is very effective when applied to mucous membranes.

"Xylocaine" (Astra-Hewlett) Ointment contains 5 per cent Lignocaine in a water-miscible basis. It is also available as a spray. "Xylodase" contains hyaluronidase in addition.

"Xylotox" (Willows Francis) Ointment contains 5 per cent of Lignocaine in a water-miscible basis.

Mepivicaine Hydrochloride syn. Carbocaine Hydrochloride (Winthrop) is a white powder, freely soluble in water and in methyl alcohol. It has an action similar to that of Lignocaine but of longer duration.

"Scandicaine" (Pharmaceutical Mfg. Co.), Mepivicaine Hydrochloride (without Adrenaline) available as 1 per cent solution in cartridges of 1·8 ml.

Prilocaine Hydrochloride is a white powder readily soluble in water and alcohol. It is said to have a quick and long lasting local anaesthetic action. It is less toxic than lignocaine. (See also **Analgesics Local** page 145.)

MACROGOLS

Macrogols syn. Polyethylene glycols are mixtures of condensation polymers of ethylene oxide and water.

The molecular weight of the polymers varies from 200 to several thousand. Polymers with molecular weights between 200 and 700 are liquid at normal temperatures. Polymers with molecular weights of over 1,000 are solids of increasing hardness as the molecular weight increases. The concept of increasing viscosity or hardness with increasing molecular weight applies also to the paraffins and alcohols. However, it should be noted that whereas the paraffin and alcohol series are different chemicals the macrogols are polymers.

The macrogols are incompatible with phenol, iodine, tannic acid and the salts of mercury and silver. Penicillin and bacitracin are rapidly inactivated by macrogols.

The macrogols are strongly hydrophilic compounds and are non-irritant to the skin, emollient and are well absorbed. They therefore make good water-miscible bases for ointments particularly where penetration of the skin is desired. Macrogols are also used as solvents for drugs such as Hydrocortisone, Undecenoic acid and Salicylic acid which are not very soluble in water. Because of the good penetration of the macrogols, the concentrations of drugs such as these in a basis of macrogols may have to be reduced.

Macrogol Ointment (Unguentum Macrogolis) B.P.C. contains equal parts of macrogol 300 and macrogol 4000 and it is used as a base.

Cetomacrogol 1000 (Cetomacrogol) B.P.C. is a macrogol ether containing 20–40 oxyethylene groups in the polyoxyethylene chain. It is a cream-coloured waxy mass that is soluble in water, acetone and alcohol.

Cetomacrogol 1000 is used in the preparation of Cetomacrogol Emulsifying Wax which can be employed for making oil-in-water emulsions that are stable over a wide pH range.

Cetomacrogol Emulsifying Ointment (Unguentum Cetomagrolis Emulsificans) B.P.C. is a mixture of Cetomacrogol Emulsifying Wax 30 per cent, Liquid Paraffin 20 per cent and White Soft Paraffin 50 per cent.

Cetomacrogol Emulsifying Wax (Cera Cetomagrolis Emulsificans) B.P.C. is obtained by melting together 2 parts of Cetomacrogol 1000 and 8 parts of Cetostearyl Alcohol.

MAGENTA

Magenta *(Magenta)* B.P.C. syn. Fuchsine is one of the group of dyestuffs obtained from coal tar. It occurs as iridescent dark green crystals consisting of a mixture of para-rosaniline (the hydrochloride of triaminotriphenyl carbinol anhydride) and rosaniline (the hydrochloride of triaminodiphenyl carbinol anhydride). It is soluble in water and in Alcohol (90 per cent) giving a deep red solution. It is incompatible with oxidizing and reducing agents.

Magenta is active against Gram-positive organisms.

Magenta Paint (*Pigmentum Magentae*) B.P.C. syn. Castellani's Paint contains 0·4 per cent of Magenta, 4 per cent of Phenol, 0·8 per cent of Boric Acid, 8 per cent of Resorcinol in 4 per cent of Acetone, 8·5 per cent of Alcohol (90 per cent) and water to 100 per cent.

This paint may be applied to fungal infections of the skin. It should be used cautiously at first. It is not effective in cases of onychomycosis. The affected area should be painted every two or three days. As the dye tends to come off the skin, precautions should be taken to avoid staining clothing and bed linen.

MAGNESIUM

Magnesium Sulphate (*Magnesii Sulphas*) B.P. syn. Epsom Salts, $MgSO_4 \cdot 7H_2O$, occurs as colourless crystals with a saline, bitter taste containing not less than 99·5 per cent $MgSO_4$ when dried to a constant weight at 300° C. Magnesium Sulphate is readily soluble in water and is sparingly soluble in alcohol.

Magnesium sulphate when dissolved in fairly high concentrations in water exerts an osmotic action. Magnesium Sulphate Paste is hygroscopic, induces a local hyperaemia and has a slight anaesthetic action. Magnesium sulphate is popular and sound for home use in a foot-bath, relieving congestion and soothing sore and tender feet. Magnesium Sulphate Paste may be used in the treatment of septic conditions such as onychia and paronychia and infected cavities generally. If the paste is freshly prepared by the operator from magnesium sulphate and glycerin, care should be taken to see that the paste is smooth and not gritty. Exsiccated magnesium sulphate and not the crystals should be used. Magnesium Sulphate Paste, however, is not easy to prepare and should, where possible, be prepared by a pharmacist.

Magnesium Sulphate Paste (*Pasta Magnesii Sulphatis*) B.P.C. syn. Morison's Paste contains 45 per cent of Exsiccated Magnesium Sulphate, 0·5 per cent of Phenol in Glycerin to 100 per cent.

MALACHITE GREEN (see Brilliant Green)

MALIC ACID (see Acetic Acid)

MENTHOL

Menthol (*Menthol*) B.P. is *p*-methan-3-ol $CH_3 \cdot C_6H_9(OH) \cdot C_3H_7$

and is a white crystalline substance which is readily soluble in alcohol and ether, but is only sparingly soluble in water. It has a characteristic peppermint smell.

Menthol is antiseptic and analgesic and when applied to the skin it relieves pain, stimulates the nerve endings of cold, dilates the superficial blood vessels and has a rubefacient action. It is generally used in conjunction with other ingredients in rubefacient ointments. Foot-powders may include 2 per cent of menthol for its cooling effect.

Menthol is an ingredient of Methyl Salicylate Ointment, Compound which contains 10 per cent of menthol (see Methyl Salicylate).

MEPIVACAINE (see Lignocaine)

MERCURY

A number of different compounds of mercury, both inorganic and organic, may be used externally, and the metal itself may be triturated with chalk or with fats for external use. Formerly the inorganic compounds were widely used in the treatment of syphilis and of mycotic or bacterial skin infections. The use of mercury externally in syphilis is now obsolete and the use of the inorganic compounds for skin infections has been largely replaced by the employment of the organic compounds which are less irritant.

Mercury compounds are incompatible with iodine and the iodides.

Mercury Ointment Compound (*Unguentum Hydrargyri Compositum*) B.P.C. 1959 contains the equivalent of 12 per cent of Mercury and consists of Mercury Ointment B.P. 1959 (which contains 30 per cent of Mercury) 40 per cent, Yellow Beeswax 24 per cent, Olive Oil 24 per cent and Flowers of Camphor 12 per cent.

This preparation is commonly, but erroneously, called Scott's Dressing: Scott's Dressing is a particular method of applying Compound Ointment of Mercury to the knee.

Compound Ointment of Mercury is indicated for chronic synovitis and for chronic and subacute bursitis in order to promote the absorption of the inflammatory exudate. The ointment is applied spread on lint and should be left in position for 24 hours only.

Phenylmercuric Nitrate (*Phenylhydragyri Nitas*) B.P. is a white powder containing not less than 98 per cent of:
$$C_6H_5 \cdot HgOH, C_6H_5 \cdot HgNO_3$$
It is soluble 1 part in 1,500 parts of water and 1 in 1,000 of alcohol (95 per cent).

Phenylmercuric nitrate is a non-irritant bacteriostatic and fungicide. Its activity is slightly reduced in the presence of body fluids. A 1 in 1,000 solution in isopropyl alcohol is used for mycotic infections or a 1 in 1,500 solution as a bacteriostatic. Phenylmercuric nitrate is widely used in fungicidal creams, ointments and dusting-powders. Phenylmercuric acetate has the advantage of being slightly more soluble than the nitrate.

"Polycrest Cream" (Clinical Products) contains 0·25 per cent Phenylmercuric Nitrate with Amethocaine Hydrochloride and Benzocaine. It is an antipruritic and fungicidal cream.

Phenylmercuric Acetate (*Phenylhydrargyri Acetas*) B.P.C. is a white powder containing not less than 98 per cent of:

$$C_6H_5 \cdot HgO \cdot CO \cdot CH_3$$

It is soluble slowly 1 part in 600 parts of water and is soluble in acetone and alcohol. It may be used in lieu of Phenyl Mercuric Nitrate.

"Phytodermine Cream" (May & Baker) contains Phenylmercuric Acetate, Salicylic Acid and Terpineol.

(N.B. "Phytodermine Powder" contains no Phenylmercuric Acetate.)

Thiomersal (*Thiomersalum*) B.P. syn. Thiomersalate,

$$C_2H_5 \cdot Hg \cdot S \cdot C_6H_4 \cdot COONa$$

is the sodium salt of ethyl mercurithiosalicylic acid. It is a cream-coloured crystalline powder, soluble in water and alcohol. A 1:1,000 isotonic solution is used as an antiseptic. It is effective against certain non-sporing organisms. As a fungicide it is used 1:1,000 in a cream base.

"Merthiolate" (Eli Lilley) contains Thiomersalate 1:1,000 in an Alcohol-acetone-aqueous solution.

"Metaphen" (Abbot Laboratories) is Nitromersol (U.S.N.F.), Anhydro-2-hydroxymercuri-6-methyl-3-nitrophenol, dissolved in NaOH, when it forms the sodium salt. A 1:2,500 solution is used as a paint for infected skin conditions, for small wounds and for skin sterilization.

Hydrargaphen is a complex phenylmercuric salt. It is a bacteriostatic agent effective against Gram-positive and Gram-negative bacteria. It also inhibits the growth of some pathogenic fungi, including *Trichophyton* spp., *Epidermophyton* and *Candida* spp.

"Penofome" (Ward, Blenkinsop) contains 0·4 per cent of Hydrargaphen in a detergent base and is used as a preoperative skin-cleansing agent.

"Penotrane" (Ward, Blenkinsop) may be obtained as a 0·1 per

cent aqueous solution of Hydrargaphen or as a 0·4 per cent dusting-powder. "Penotrane" is also available as a jelly and tincture.

METHARGEN (see Silver)

METHYL ALCOHOL (see Alcohols)

METHYL SALICYLATE

Methyl Salicylate (*Methylis Salicylas*) B.P. is a colourless liquid, with a characteristic wintergreen odour, containing not less than 99·0 per cent of $C_6H_4 \cdot OH \cdot COOCH_3$. It is slightly soluble in water and is miscible with alcohol (90 per cent), with ether and with chloroform.

Methyl salicylate is analgesic, slightly antiseptic and is a powerful rubefacient.

Methyl salicylate is most effective when applied in conjunction with heat although it is still very effective when applied without. It is indicated in all types of aseptic inflammation where the skin is not broken and where a penetrating rubefacient is required. Methyl salicylate relieves congestion and muscle pain. It may also be used in the treatment of heavy plantar callus, being rubbed in after the removal of the callus, in order to stimulate the peripheral circulation. Adhesive padding and strapping is contra-indicated after the use of methyl salicylate because it may cause maceration. Methyl salicylate is one of the most popular and effective rubefacients for external use. It is frequently used combined with Iodine Ointment, Non-staining and with Iodine Oil.

Methyl Salicylate Liniment (*Linimentum Methylis Salicylatis*, B.P.C. contains 25 per cent of Methyl Salicylate in Arachis Oil or Cottonseed Oil to 100 per cent.

Methyl Salicylate and Eucalyptus Liniment (*Linimentum Methylis Salicylatis et Eucalypti*) B.P.C. 1954 contains 5 per cent of Menthol, 10 per cent of Oil of Eucalyptus, 25 per cent of Rectified Oil of Camphor with Methyl Salicylate to 100 per cent.

Iodine Ointment non-staining, with Methyl Salicylate (*Unguentum Iodi Denigrescens cum Methylis Salicylatis*) B.P.C. contains 5 per cent of Methyl Salicylate in Iodine Ointment, Non-staining, to 100 per cent.

Methyl Salicylate Ointment (*Unguentum Methylis Salicylatis*) B.P.C. contains 50 per cent of Methyl Salicylate in 25 per cent of White Beeswax and 25 per cent of Hydrous Wool Fat.

Methyl Salicylate Ointment, Compound (*Unguentum Methylis*

Salicylatis Compositum) B.P.C. contains 50 per cent of Methyl Salicylate, 10 per cent of Menthol, 2·5 per cent of Eucalyptol, 2·5 per cent of Cajuput Oil, in 20 per cent of White Beeswax and 15 per cent of Hydrous Wool Fat.

"Analgesic Balm" (Parke, Davis), "Balmosa" (Oppenheimer), "Bengue's Balsam" (Bengue's), are proprietary preparations which are similar to Methyl Salicylate Ointment, Compound.

"Radian-A" (Radiol Co.) is a rubefacient paint containing, among its active ingredients, 21·3 per cent of Methyl Salicylate.

MONOCHLOROACETIC ACID

Monochloroacetic Acid $CH_2Cl \cdot COOH$, occurs as deliquescent crystals which are readily soluble in water, alcohol and ether.

Monochloroacetic acid is caustic and may be used in the treatment of warts.

The Treatment of Warts with Monochloroacetic Acid

Method 1. The use of Monochloroactic Acid by itself.

(a) After removing the superficial layers of the growth, the wart is soaked with a saturated solution of monochloroacetic acid. The return period is 3–14 days, generally 7 days.

(b) After removing the superficial layers of the wart a crystal of monochloroacetic acid is gently rubbed into the growth for a timed period. The dosage will vary according to the duration of the application, 30–60 seconds is suggested as an experimental starting point. The return period is 3–14 days, generally 7 days.

In both the above treatments the foot must be kept out of water in the intervals between treatments.

Method I is indicated as a treatment for large single growths, or for "mother" growths, when there is plenty of adipose tissue between the wart and the bone. It is likely that a breakdown will be produced and there may be some pain. The method is contra-indicated when breakdown is to be avoided.

Method II. (Used in conjunction with Salicylic Acid.)

(a) After proceeding as in Method I (a) or I (b) above, the wart is dressed with a standard wart ointment dressing using 60 per cent salicylic acid ointment. The return period is 5–7 days.

(b) A standard wart dressing using 60 per cent salicylic acid ointment is applied and a small crystal of monochloroacetic acid is pushed well into the ointment so that it lies in contact with the growth. The return period is 5–7 days.

In both (a) and (b) above the foot must be kept out of water. Method II is indicated as a treatment for large, obstinate growths rather than as an initial treatment. It is contra-indicated when break-down is to be avoided.

To neutralize or to stop the action of monochloroacetic acid, first dilute with plenty of water and then give a foot-bath containing sodium bicarbonate. Potassium Hydroxide Solution may be used instead of sodium bicarbonate but it must be rinsed off afterwards.

NEOMYCIN SULPHATE (see Antibiotics)

NITRIC ACID

Nitric Acid (*Acidum Nitricum*) B.P. is a colourless liquid which fumes on exposure to air. It contains 70 per cent of HNO_3. Nitric acid should be stored in glass-stoppered bottles and should never be kept in the same cupboard as instruments, nail burrs or other metal objects.

Nitric acid is caustic with a powerful oxidizing action. It is used for the treatment of warts and occasionally of vascular corns and hyper-granulation tissue. It is a powerful caustic on account of its oxidizing power and because it coagulates proteins.

The Treatment of Warts with Nitric Acid

Method I. After the removal of the superficial layers of the wart, nitric acid is applied to the wart using a glass rod, or a wooden applicator wrapped round with a *very little* cotton wool. The acid is left on the wart for about five minutes and its action is then stopped by means of a 10 per cent solution of phenol. The skin will be stained a bright yellow owing to the formation of trinitrophenol. The phenol will also serve to reduce the pain caused by the action of the nitric acid.

Method II. After operating, the growth is first saturated with 5 per cent phenol for 5 minutes. Then an excess of nitric acid is applied to the wart and left on for 20–30 seconds. The growth is again saturated with 5 per cent phenol. This method obviates much of the pain which might otherwise be caused by the nitric acid.

In both these methods each application is complete in itself and they are good methods to use where rapid results are required and treatment may have to be interrupted.

Two things should be particularly noted with regard to nitric acid:

(i) Because it fumes when exposed to the air, it has the appearance of being a very strong acid and it may frighten nervous patients.

(ii) Owing to its oxidizing action, it has a very superficial action on the skin when it is applied in small doses.

NYSTATIN (see Antibiotics)

OILS, ESSENTIAL

Clove Oil (*Oleum Caryophylli*) B.P. is distilled from the unopened buds of *Eugenia aromatica*. It contains from 85–90 per cent of eugenol $OH \cdot OCH_3 \cdot C_6H_3 \cdot CH_2 \cdot CH:CH_2$. Clove oil has rubefacient and analgesic properties and may be used externally on chilblains and rheumatic conditions. It is used generally as an ingredient of a compound oil or ointment, or may be diluted 1 part to 3 parts of olive oil for application to chilblains and neuralgic conditions.

Eucalyptus Oil (*Oleum Eucalypti*) B.P. is distilled from the fresh leaves of various species of Eucalyptus. It contains not less than 70 per cent of cineole $C_{10}H_{18}O$. Eucalyptus oil is analgesic, antiseptic and healing and may be used on broken chilblains, combined with white soft paraffin. Mixed with an equal quantity of olive oil, eucalyptus oil may be used as a rubefacient.

Peppermint Oil (*Oleum Mentha Piperita*) B.P. is distilled from the fresh flowing tips of *Mentha piperita* and contains not less than 45 per cent of free menthol. Peppermint oil is rubefacient and analgesic and is an ingredient of Kaolin Poultice.

Turpentine Oil (*Oleum Terebinthinae*) B.P. is distilled from oleoresin turpentine obtained from *Pinus sylvestris* and other species of Pine.

Turpentine is employed externally as a rubefacient and is an ingredient of many rubefacient liniments. Liniments containing turpentine are usually rubbed into the skin. If they are applied as dressings their action is very drastic. Stoups containing turpentine were a very ancient method of blistering when this was a common practice in medicine.

Turpentine Liniment (*Linimentum Terebinthinae*) B.P. contains 65 per cent of Turpentine Oil, with 7·5 per cent of Soft Soap, 5 per cent of Camphor and 22·5 per cent of Distilled Water.

White Liniment (*Linimentum Album*) B.P.C. 8·33 per cent Oleic Acid, 4·5 per cent Dilute Solution of Ammonia, 1·25 per cent of Ammonium Chloride, 25 per cent of Turpentine Oil in water to 100 per cent.

Rue Oil is distilled from *Ruta graveolens*. *Lotio Ruta Graveolens* is a solution of Rue Oil in spirit soap base. It is useful for nail packs because, when used with Amadou, Felt and the like, it makes a more pliable dressing than does Compound Benzoin Tincture.

OILS, EXPRESSED

There is still a number of these used in chiropody, although those such as Almond Oil, Arachis Oil, Castor Oil, Olive Oil, etc., which used to be applied as emollients, have been largely superseded by the water-containing creams.

These oils, however, are sometimes used as vehicles for medicaments. Linseed Oil is reputed to have analgesic properties, and Wheat Germ Oil (source of vitamin E) is said to break down fibrous tissue, although there seems to be no objective evidence of this.

PARAFFINS

The paraffins, like the Alcohols, are a group of substances related by a common formula C_nH_{2n+2}, e.g. CH_4, C_2H_6, C_4H_{10}, C_8H_{18}, etc. In the first members of the series, where "n" is small the Paraffins are gases at normal temperatures; as "n" increases, the members of the series become liquids, soft solids and finally very hard solids as the molecular weight increases.

Hard Paraffin (*Paraffinum Durum*) B.P. is a mixture of several of the harder members of the paraffin series of hydrocarbons in the range $C_{21}H_{44}$ to $C_{30}H_{62}$. It has a melting point of 50–57° C.

Paraffin wax is principally used in ointment bases to raise the melting point of the ointment, but may also be employed as a sterile dressing for chilblains and ulcers, e.g. "Paraffin No. 7", which consists of 25 per cent of Soft Paraffin, 10 per cent of Olive Oil, 55 per cent of Hard Paraffin, 1 per cent of Resorcinol and 2 per cent of Eucalyptus Oil. Hard Paraffin is an ingredient of Wool Alcohols Ointment, Paraffin Ointment and Simple Ointment, see under Soft Paraffin below

Liquid Paraffin (*Paraffinum Liquidum*) B.P. is a clear oily liquid obtained from petroleum after the more volatile portion has been removed by distillation. Liquid paraffin is a poor emollient. It is used for dispensing as a vehicle for other medicaments, and in the preparation of ointment and cream bases.

Soft Paraffin (*Paraffinum Molle*) B.P. syn. Yellow Soft Paraffin is a mixture of the semi-solid members of the paraffin series of hydrocarbons in the range of $C_{15}H_{32}$ to $C_{20}H_{42}$. It has a melting point of 38–56° C. "Vaseline" is a trade name of yellow soft paraffin. White soft paraffin has been bleached.

Soft paraffin is not easily absorbed by the skin and is useful as an ointment base where a surface action is required. It may be used as a sterile dressing in the form of Tulle Gras.

The following preparations are widely used as ointment bases:

Emulsifying Ointment (*Unguentum Emulsificans*) B.P. which is 30 per cent of Emulsifying Wax with 50 per cent of White Soft Paraffin and 20 per cent of Liquid Paraffin.

Aqueous Cream B.P. syn. Simple Cream which is 30 per cent of Emulsifying Ointment, 0·1 per cent of Chlorocresol with water to 100 per cent.

Wool Alcohols Ointment (*Unguentum Alcoholium Lanae*) B.P. which is 6 per cent of Wool Alcohols, 24 per cent of Hard Paraffin, 10 per cent White or Yellow Soft Paraffin with 60 per cent of Liquid Paraffin.

Paraffin Ointment (*Unguentum Paraffini*) B.P. which is 2 per cent of Beeswax, 3 per cent of Hard Paraffin, 5 per cent of Cetostearyl Alcohol with 90 per cent of White or Yellow Soft Paraffin.

Simple Ointment (*Unguentum Simplex*) B.P. which is 5 per cent of Wool Fat, 5 per cent of Hard Paraffin, 5 per cent of Cetostearyl Alcohol with 85 per cent of White or Yellow Soft Paraffin.

PARAHYDROXYBENZOIC ACID (see Salicylic Acid)

PECILOCIN (see Antibiotics)

PERU BALSAM

Peru Balsam (*Balsamum Peruvianum*) B.P.C. is a viscid brown liquid obtained from the trunk of *Myroxylon pereirae* after it has been beaten and scorched. Peru balsam is soluble in chloroform, ether and alcohol but is insoluble in water. Peru balsam is antiseptic, healing and fungicidal, and it stimulates the formation of granulation tissue in the healing process. There are now no official preparations containing Peru balsam but an ointment containing 12½ per cent of Peru balsam in a Simple Ointment base may be used in treating the breakdown of a wart after treatment with acids, in the treatment of ulcers and broken chilblains and in the treatment of heel fissures where fungal infection is suspected as a complication. A preparation containing equal parts of Peru balsam and castor oil may be used instead of the ointment. Peru balsam was used as an antiseptic in Paraffin Gauze Dressing. Continued application of Peru Balsam may cause sensitization.

PHENOL

Phenol (*Phenol*) B.P. syn. Carbolic Acid is hydroxybenzene and occurs as colourless needle-shaped, deliquescent crystals which become pinkish on keeping, and which contain not less than 98 per cent of C_6H_5OH. Phenol should be stored in a cool, dark place.

One hundred parts of phenol are liquefied by 10 parts of water and will dissolve 30–40 parts of water. As water is added to phenol, two layers are formed, one a solution of phenol in water and the other a solution of water in phenol (see Solution, page 3) until, when 1,200 parts of water have been added to the 100 parts of phenol, the phenol will be completely dissolved in the water. Phenol is also soluble 6 parts in 1 part Alcohol, 5 in 1 of Ether, 3 in 1 of Glycerin and 1 in 200 of Liquid Paraffin. Phenol is soluble in fats.

Phenol is incompatible with the salts of iron. When phenol (a solid) is mixed with camphor, menthol, thymol or chloral hydrate (which are also solids) the two solids liquefy.

Phenol was the original choice of antiseptic made by Lister in his early work on aseptic technique but, since it is as toxic to tissue cells as it is to bacteria, its popularity as an antiseptic has declined. Solutions of phenol 0·2 to 1 per cent in water are bacteriostatic and solutions of phenol 2·5 to 5 per cent are bactericidal. The antiseptic and germicidal properties of phenol vary considerably with the base in which phenol is dispensed. Phenol has little or no germicidal activity in alcohol, in oil or in purely fatty bases. This is shown by the fact that ointments of phenol may become rancid. Sodium chloride increases the activity of phenol by reducing its solubility in water and increasing the concentration of phenol in contact with the bacterial organisms.

Phenol is also analgesic and caustic and must always be used with care (*a*) owing to its caustic properties, and (*b*) due to the fact that it causes constriction of the smaller blood vessels when applied as a wet dressing and tends, on account of its analgesic properties, to cause a painless gangrene. Phenol paralyzes the sensory nerve endings in the skin and is used as an analgesic in cases of pruritis and also, on occasions, to alleviate the pain when operating on a hard corn. In the latter case it is less effective than a sound operating technique.

Phenol Glycerin (*Glycerinum Phenolis*) B.P.C. contains 16 per cent of Phenol in Glycerin to 100 per cent.

Liquefied Phenol (*Phenol Liquefactum*) B.P. contains 80 per cent of Phenol with water to 100 per cent. It is a solution of water in phenol.

Indications for using Phenol

A 5 per cent solution of phenol in water may be applied to a painful corn by a swab soaked in the solution, for about 5 minutes, the sac is then washed out well with spirit. This treatment is particularly useful where the sac is soggy and macerated. On warts, phenol may be used in conjunction with nitric acid (see page 194) or the growth may be saturated with Liquefied Phenol and left for 4 days when the patient should return for the removal of the dead tissue and for further treatment. This is a useful treatment for a very painful wart and also where much maceration has been caused by the use of salicylic acid or of pyrogallol.

Liquefied Phenol in water may be painted on to heavy, macerated callus. It may also be used as a caustic for nail work.

Liquefied Phenol may be employed in the cold sterilization of instruments, the instruments, being immersed in it for 10 minutes and then in alcohol for 5 minutes.

Phenol 25 per cent with Camphor 75 per cent may be used as a fungicidal paint.

Burns on the skin caused by phenol, or phenol dropped accidentally on the skin, should be swabbed with spirit or glycerin, either of which readily dissolves phenol.

PHENOXYETHANOL

Phenoxyethanol (*Phenoxyethanol*) B.P.C. Trade name: "Phenoxetol" (Nipa) is 2-phenoxyethanol: $C_6H_5O \cdot CH_2 \cdot CH_2OH$ It is a slightly viscous, colourless liquid, which is soluble in water and miscible with alcohol, ether and acetone.

Phenoxyethanol is an antiseptic which has a selective action against Gram-negative organisms and especially against *Pseudomonas pyocyanea*. It may be used as a 2 per cent aqueous solution or as a 2 per cent cream, where infection with *Ps. pyocyanea* is suspected. Phenoxyethanol is also used locally in conjunction with other antiseptics, such as the acridines, cetrimide, penicillin and the sulphonamides, in order to reinforce their action against Gram-negative organisms.

"Phytocil Cream" (Wade Pharmaceuticals) contains 2 per cent 3-phenoxypropanol and 1 per cent chlorophenoxyethanol with Salicylic Acid and Menthol. It is used for the treatment of dermatomycoses. A dusting-powder is also obtainable.

PHENYLMERCURIC ACETATE, NITRATE (see Mercury)

PODOPHYLLUM RESIN

Podophyllum Resin (*Podophylli Resinae*) B.P. syn. Podophyllin is a mixture of resins obtained from the dried rhizome and roots of *Podophyllum pelatum* or *P. hexandrum*. It is a light brown amorphous powder. Since it is very irritant to the eyes care should be taken when the powder is being handled.

Podophyllin ointment may be used in the treatment of superficial groups of warts, or a solution of 10 per cent of Podophyllum Resin in ethyl or isopropyl alcohol may be used for the same purpose. The solution may be applied daily by the patient.

Podophyllin Paint, Compound (*Pigmentum Podophyllini*) B.P.C. contains 15 per cent of Podophyllum Resin in Compound Benzoin Tincture to 100 per cent.

"Posalfilin" (Camden Chemical Co.) contains 20 per cent of Podophyllin and 25 per cent of Salicylic Acid. This has proved successful in a number of cases of mosaic or large warts. The ointment is rubbed into the growth and covered with waterproof strapping. The return period is from 3–7 days.

"Vericap SAP" (Cuxon, Gerrard). Self-adhesive plasters in two sizes, medicated with an ointment containing 20 per cent of Podophyllum Resin and 25 per cent of Salicylic Acid. Protective felt rings are incorporated in the dressing. They are used for the treatment of warts. "Vericap PLL" consists of elastic adhesive plaster medicated with an ointment containing 20 per cent of Podophyllum Resin and 20 per cent of Linseed Oil, also with protective felt rings.

POLYNOXYLIN

Polynoxylin is a condensation product of formaldehyde and urea. It is an amorphous white powder which is relatively insoluble in water. It does not liberate free formaldehyde.

"Ponoxylan Gel" (Berk Pharmaceuticals Ltd.) contains 10 per cent Polynoxylin in a basis of polythene glycol polymers containing 5 per cent water.

It has an anti-bacterial action against all common pathogens, both Gram-positive and Gram-negative and strains resistant to antibiotics and sulphonamides. No strains resistant to Ponoxylan have been produced under trial. "Ponoxylan Gel" is also anti-inflammatory and antipruritic. Its action is said to resemble that of the corticosteroids. It cannot be absorbed systemically and its use is therefore restricted to topical application. Its action is enhanced in the presence of pus and serum, and it is non-toxic.

"Ponoxylan Gel" has been proved particularly useful in the treatment of ulceration by eliminating sloughs and promoting healing. The area should be cleansed with saline solution if necessary and the "Ponoxylan Gel" applied on sterile non-adherent gauze. The maximum return period should be 2 days. Initially daily dressings are desirable.

"Ponoxylan Derm" (West-Silten) contains 5 per cent Polynoxylin in a soapless basis.

"Anaflex" (Geistlich) contains 10 per cent Polynoxylin as a cream or as a paste.

POTASSIUM SALTS

Potassium Hydroxide (*Potassii Hydroxidi*) B.P. syn. Caustic Potash occurs as white deliquescent cakes or pellets containing not less than 85 per cent of KOH. It is readily soluble in water and alcohol.

Potassium Hydroxide may be used as a caustic for warts using the following technique:

1. The superficial layers of the wart are pared away with the knife.

2. The foot is immersed in a warm foot-bath of plain water for 5 minutes. Some operators omit this step and rub the pellet of KOH into the dry lesion.

3. The foot is then dried and a pellet of KOH is rubbed gently into the growth. The pellet may conveniently be held in a wooden holder made from a clothes peg.

4. The foot is again immersed in the foot-bath for about two minutes.

5. Following this immersion, a jelly-like material will be found to have formed over the wart. This is scraped away.

6. Glacial Acetic Acid is applied to the growth.

There is no return period because each application is complete in itself.

Potassium Hydroxide Solution (*Liquor Potassii Hydroxidi*) B.P. is an aqueous solution of Potassium Hydroxide containing 5 per cent of KOH. It may be employed in order to soften very hard corns, onychophosis, nails, callus, etc. It is generally applied as a swab saturated with the Potassium Hydroxide Solution, which is left in place for about five minutes before operating. The tissues should always be washed free from the alkali after operating. Potassium Hydroxide Solution should be stored in a container having a rubber stopper.

Potassium Hydroxyquinoline Sulphate (*Potassii Hydroxyquinolini*

202 AN INTRODUCTION TO THERAPEUTICS FOR CHIROPODISTS

Sulphas) B.P.C. consists of a mixture of potassium sulphate and 8-hydroxyquinoline sulphate (C_9H_6[OH]N)$_2$,H_2SO_4 containing about the equivalent of 50 per cent of 8-hydroxyquinoline. It is a light powder of crystalline nature which is soluble in water, and sparingly soluble in alcohol. Potassium hydroxyquinoline sulphate is incompatible with ferric salts and with bismuth.

Potassium hydroxyquinoline sulphate is a powerful germicide and deodorant. It may be used as aqueous solution in strengths of 1:2,000 to 1:500 for skin infections and the 1:2,000 solution may be applied frequently to mycotic infections. This solution may also be used as a lotion in the treatment of hyperidrosis and bromidrosis.

Potassium Permanganate (*Potassii Permanganas*) B.P. occurs as deep purple crystals containing not less than 99·0 per cent of $KMnO_4$. It is soluble 1 part in 16 parts of water.

Potassium permanganate is incompatible with glycerin, alcohol, fats, oils and all vegetable oxidizable matter, with ammonia, ammonium salts, iodine and with Hydrogen Peroxide Solution.

Solution tablets of potassium permanganate are available.

Potassium permanganate is an active antiseptic on account of its oxidizing action. Solutions of potassium permanganate tend to stain the skin brown and the stain may be removed with very dilute hydrochloric acid. Potassium permanganate is also deodorant and fungicidal.

Potassium permanganate may be used in a foot-bath in the surgery or for the home treatment of hyperidrosis and bromidrosis and also for septic conditions. Sufficient crystals are added to the water in the foot-bath to tinge the water pink. The crystals dissolve very slowly and time must be allowed for complete solution to take place. Five or six crystals to 2½ litres (½ a gallon) of water are sufficient. Potassium permanganate may also be used in the form of a 1 per cent aqueous solution as a paint for hyperidrosis and bromidrosis, the paint being applied once weekly.

POVIDONE-IODINE (see Iodine)

PRILOCAINE (see Lignocaine)

PROFLAVINE (see Amino-acridines)

PROPIONIC ACID

Propionic Acid (*Acidum Propionicum*) B.P.C. 1954 occurs as a colourless liquid containing not less than 99 per cent of C_2H_5·COOH. It is miscible with water, alcohol and ether.

Propionic acid and its salts are used as fungicides either as ointments containing from 2·5 to 3·5 per cent of the acid or in dusting-powders containing 0·25 per cent of the acid. The zinc salt of propionic acid is frequently incorporated in preparations containing the acid.

PYROGALLOL

Pyrogallol syn. Pyrogallic Acid is benzene 1-, 2-, 3-triol $C_6H_3(OH)_3$. It occurs either as light feathery crystals or dense hard crystals, either form becoming discoloured on exposure to the air. Pyrogallol has a strong affinity for oxygen and is a powerful reducing agent.

Pyrogallol is caustic and analgesic and it is interesting to compare the formulae for:

Phenol   Resorcinol and Pyrogallol

Pyrogallol is used in dermatology in ointment form in strengths varying from 2–10 per cent for the treatment of psoriasis, lupus vulgaris and mycotic infections. In chiropody it is more generally used as a caustic for vascular corns, neurovascular corns and warts. Pyrogallol has an analgesic action and is therefore indicated as a caustic for the more painful types of lesion. On vascular corns and neurovascular corns it is used in the form of a 20 per cent ointment and on warts as a 40 per cent ointment. In both cases the ointment is applied in the routine manner. The return period is from 4–14 days but is generally 7 days. Pyrogallic plasters in strengths from 10–40 per cent are used in the treatment of plantar callus, especially of the vascular type.

Pyrogallol produces a very dark brown, matt eschar, which is white in the deeper layers. In general, pyrogallol has the reputation of being a milder escharotic than salicylic acid but it must be remembered that the action of pyrogallol is cumulative. If small quantities are used then the action of the pyrogallol is quite mild, but if large quantities are used, or if the medicament is used over long periods, it must be borne in mind that, once an undetermined time and/or quantity of pyrogallol has been reached, the action of the pyrogallol becomes very drastic indeed and a very severe breakdown of tissues may be produced. The quantity of the medicament in the 40 per cent plaster is not sufficient to cause very drastic effects so that there is a marked contrast between the action of the 40 per cent plaster and the 40 per cent ointment. The action of the pyrogallol is also continuous, that is to say the action may continue after the removal of the coagulum produced by pyrogallol even though fresh quantities are not applied. In general, ointments of pyrogallol should be used only for short series of treatments.

Pyrogallol Ointment, either 20 per cent or 40 per cent strength mixed with an equal quantity of Wheat Germ Oil, has enjoyed a measure of popularity in the treatment of fibrous corns. The preparations are known as "WP" Ointment. The effect of the Wheat Germ Oil is problematical although it is suggested that it inhibits the formation of fibrous tissue. Wheat Germ Oil is now difficult to obtain and is very expensive.

PYROXYLIN

Pyroxylin (*Pyroxylinum*) B.P. is prepared by the action of a mixture of nitric and sulphuric acids on cotton wool, and has approximately the composition of cellulose tetranitrate $C_{12}H_{16}O_6(ONO_2)_4$.

In appearance, pyroxylin is a yellowish mass of filaments resembling raw cotton. It is soluble in a mixture of 1 volume of alcohol and 3 volumes of solvent ether, and is also soluble in acetone.

Flexible Collodion (*Collodium Flexile*) B.P. contains Pyroxylin 1·6 per cent, Colophony 3 per cent, Castor Oil 2 per cent, Alcohol (90 per cent) 24 per cent in Solvent Ether to 100 per cent.

When Flexible Collodion is painted on to the skin, the ether and the alcohol evaporate leaving a thin film on the surface of the skin. Flexible collodion may be applied in order to coat surgically clean cuts or, combined with cotton wool, to make cocoon dressings, splints and false nails. It is also used as a vehicle for other medicaments.

Collodions made with glycerin are said to provide a more elastic and flexible film which is less likely to dry out and peel off. An example is Kelly's Paint which consists of 3 parts of Compound Benzoin Tincture, 1 part Flexible Collodion and 1 part of Glycerin.

Oxidized Cellulose (*Cellulosum Oxidatum*) B.P. may be prepared by the oxidation of cotton, usually in the form of gauze with nitrogen dioxide.

Oxidized Cellulose is an absorbable haemostatic. When applied to a bleeding surface it swells and forms a brown gelatinous mass which is absorbed in 2 to 7 days. It should be used dry.

"Oxycel" (Parke, Davis) is Oxidized Cellulose available as sterilized gauze pads.

"Surgicel" (Ethicon) is Oxidized Regenerated Cellulose and is similar to, but not identical with, Oxidized Cellulose.

SALICYLIC ACID

Salicylic Acid (*Acidum Salicylicum*) B.P. is *ortho*-hydroxybenzoic acid and is a light, feathery crystalline powder or colourless crystals containing not less than 99·5 per cent of $C_6H_4 \cdot OH \cdot COOH$. Salicylic acid is soluble 1 part in 550 parts of water, 1 in 4 of Alcohol (95 per cent) and is readily soluble in ether.

Salicylic acid is incompatible with sal volatile and it gives a deep violet colour with traces of ferric salts.

According to the strength in which it is used, salicylic acid is antiseptic, astringent (3–5 per cent in solutions and dusting-powders), fungicidal (about 5 per cent in dusting-powders and lotions) keratoplastic (up to 6 per cent) and keratolytic (above 10 per cent). Salicylic acid is not commonly used as an antiseptic *per se*, its antiseptic value is incidental to its other qualities.

Both official and unofficial preparations of salicylic acid are widely used in chiropody, and it is used also in most proprietary corn paints and wart solvents, generally combined with creosote as an analgesic.

As an astringent, salicylic acid is used as Spiritus Pedibus or as a 5 per cent solution in Industrial Methylated Spirit. Spiritus Pedibus has the advantage of being a preparation recognized by the Board of Customs and Excise and is correspondingly easier to obtain. Many dusting-powders for the feet contain from 3–5 per cent of salicylic acid for its astringent and fungicidal properties.

As a fungicide, Spiritus Pedibus may again be used but generally this is a prophylactic to be used in conjunction with some more active method of treatment. From 3–5 per cent of salicylic acid in Compound Benzoin Tincture may be used as a fungicidal paint and Compound Benzoic Acid Ointment which contains 3 per cent of salicylic acid remains one of the most effective fungicidal ointments.

Salicylic Acid Ointment and Zinc and Salicylic Acid Paste (Lassar's Paste) each contain 2 per cent of salicylic acid. These are soothing preparations which are valuable in treating inflammations of the skin.

Perhaps it is as a keratolytic that salicylic acid is most widely used in chiropody. "Keratolytic" is a better word than "caustic" to use in connection with salicylic acid, because its action is not to destroy tissues but to break down the keratinized stratum corneum and to cause it to become softened and macerated. Salicylic acid will, however, cause the destruction of non-keratinized cells.

When salicylic acid is applied to the skin in the form of an ointment, plaster or collodion containing more than 10 per cent of the acid, a white rubbery coagulum is produced. The bulk of the keratinized tissue is increased by the action of the acid. The action of salicylic acid is cumulative rather than immediate and may continue after the dressing has been removed. It is important that the coagulum produced by salicylic acid should be completely removed before fresh acid is applied, and it is also important that it should be removed within a reasonable time, say three weeks, after the preparation has been applied. If the coagulum is not removed the macerated tissue may become infected. It is for this reason that the use of corn plaster by the general public is to be deprecated. When a corn plaster is applied the hard corneous tissue is softened and macerated; it is not destroyed, but remains until the patient attempts to remove it with a razor blade. Even if the patient does not do this, the salicylic acid may have macerated the outer layers to such an extent that a portal of entry is provided for pyogenic bacteria. The same thing may still happen if the acid is applied by the chiropodist and left unattended for a long period. It cannot be too strongly emphasized that salicylic acid ointments and plasters cannot take the place of the knife, but must always be used in conjunction with careful operating to remove as much keratinized tissue or macerated coagulum as possible. When salicylic acid has been used, special care must be taken to wipe the knife clean after operating. Tissue saturated with salicylic acid, carried over to the instrument tray, does considerable damage to instruments.

Salicylic acid in an ointment base is indicated where a drastic and localized effect is required, care being taken to protect the surrounding healthy tissues. Salicylic acid ointments are used on corns and warts, and in the lower strengths on nails. Salicylic acid as a plaster or in collodion is indicated where a diffuse, mild action is required, e.g. on an area of callus. Collodion of salicylic acid is painted on and allowed to dry. Plasters of salicylic acid generally require to be strapped in place because they are not sufficiently adhesive to adhere sufficiently firmly to the skin. Salicylic acid may be dispensed in various ointment bases, e.g. Hard Paraffin 10 per cent with Soft Paraffin 90 per cent; Lanette Wax 6 per cent with Soft Paraffin 94 per cent; Ointment of Colophony as hard bases for use in summer or in warm climates; or Soft Paraffin, Macrogol Ointment or Simple Ointment in winter or in cold climates.

Indications

Ointments: 10–15 per cent may be applied to onychophosis, the return period being 7 days.

20–40 per cent may be applied to interdigital hard corns or digital hard corns and also hard corns on the plantar surface. The use of salicylic acid may be alternated with the application of silver nitrate 25 per cent solution in water or liquefied phenol to minimize maceration of the surrounding tissues. The minimum return period is 4–7 days and the maximum 3 weeks.

50, 60 and 70 per cent may be applied to warts (see Treatment of Warts, page 104).

Plasters: 10, 20 and 40 per cent may be applied to hard corns, and 20 or 40 per cent may be applied to areas of callus.

The 40 per cent plaster is sometimes applied to the "chalky" type of wart found on elderly patients.

Collodion: The official collodion, which contains 12 per cent of salicylic acid, may be used on callus, onychophosis and on hyperkeratosis of a diffuse nature such as that produced as a result of fungal infection.

Official Preparations

Salicylic Acid Collodion (Collodium Acidi Salicylici) B.P.C. contains Salicylic Acid 12 per cent in Flexible Collodion to 100 per cent.

Compound Salicylic Acid Dusting-powder (Conspersus Acidi Salicylici Compositus) B.P.C. 1963 syn. Pulvis pro Pedibus contains Salicylic Acid 3 per cent, Boric Acid 5 per cent and Purified Talc to 100 per cent. This powder must not be applied to raw or weeping surfaces.

Zinc and Salicylic Acid Dusting-powder (Conspersus Zinci Oxidi et Acidi Salicylici) B.P.C. contains Salicylic Acid 5 per cent, Zinc Oxide 20 per cent and Starch 75 per cent.

The above two dusting-powders are astringent and fungicidal and are widely used as prophylactic powders against fungal infection in cases of hyperidrosis. They are also useful as astringent powders in the active treatment of hyperidrosis and bromidrosis especially Compound Salicylic Acid Dusting-powder.

Salicylic Acid Ointment (Unguentum Acidi Salicylici) B.P. contains 2 per cent of Salicylic Acid in Ointment of Wool Alcohols to 100 per cent. This ointment is sometimes used instead of Lassar's Paste. It has a much softer base. It is important to note that this is the official Ointment of Salicylic Acid. If Salicylic Acid Ointment were to be ordered without the strength being specified, this official ointment would be supplied.

Salicylic Acid and Sulphur Ointment (Unguentum Acidi Salicylici et Sulphuris) B.P.C. contains 3 per cent of Salicylic Acid and 3 per cent of Sulphur in Hydrous Ointment to 100 per cent. It is a fungicidal and parasiticidal ointment.

Zinc Oxide with Salicylic Acid Paste (Pasta Zinci Oxidi cum Acido Salicylico) B.P. syn. Lassar's Paste, contains 2 per cent of Salicylic Acid, 24 per cent of Zinc Oxide, 24 per cent of Starch in White Soft Paraffin to 100 per cent.

This may be used as a soothing preparation to plaster rash and to similar inflammations of the skin. It is generally applied spread thinly on lint. Because it is a very stiff preparation, it does not tend to clog, and may be used where there is some exudation from a skin condition. On account of its stiffness, it may also be used as a buffer ointment.

Salicylic Acid Self-adhesive Plaster (Emplastrum Acidi Salicylici) B.P.C. contains up to 40 per cent of Salicylic Acid. A 20 per cent plaster would, however, be supplied for Salicylic Acid Plaster unless another strength were indicated.

Foot Spirit (Spiritus Pedibus) contains 3 per cent of Salicylic Acid, 0·5 per cent of Methyl Salicylate, 1 per cent of Diethyl Phthalate in Industrial Methylated Spirit. This is an astringent lotion which is also prophylactic against fungal infection. It may be recommended for daily use in cases of hyperidrosis and bromidrosis, in cases of maceration of the skin and where the skin requires hardening.

"Vericap S.A.P." (Cuxon, Gerrard). Self-adhesive plaster, medicated with an ointment containing 25 per cent of Salicylic Acid and Podophyllum Resin. For the treatment of warts.

Parahydroxybenzoic Acid is a close chemical relative of salicylic acid, differing from it only in the relative positions of the —OH and —COOH radicles in the benzene ring.

Ortho-hydroxybenzoic Acid   *Para*-hydroxybenzoic Acid
Salicylic Acid

Parahydroxybenzoic acid produces a drier and less rubbery

coagulum than salicylic acid and appears to cause less maceration of the surrounding tissues. It may be used instead of salicylic acid in the treatment of corns and warts in the same strengths as salicylic acid. It does not appear to cause a breakdown of tissue in the same way as salicylic acid may do when used to treat warts.

"Catox" (Harker, Stagg) is a cream containing 3·1 per cent of salicylic acid with cetyl-alcohol tar distillate and sulphur in a water-miscible basis. For dermatomycosis.

"Monphytol" (Laboratories for Applied Biology) contains 1·2 per cent salicylic acid, with boric acid, chlorbutol and undecenoic acid. For the treatment of obstinate dermatomycosis.

"Phytodermine Cream" (May & Baker) contains 3 per cent salicylic acid with phenyl mercuric acetate. "Phytodermine Powder" contains 5 per cent of Salicylic Acid and 5 per cent of Methyl hydroxybenzoate.

SCARLET RED

Scarlet Red (*Rubrum Scarlatinum*) B.P.C. 1959 syn. Biebrich Scarlet is 1-[*p*-(*o*-Tolylazo)-*o*-tolylazo]naphth-2-ol:

$$CH_3·C_6H_4N:NC_6H_3N:N·C_{10}H_5OH$$

It is a dark brownish-red powder, soluble in oils and fats but insoluble in water.

Scarlet red is a healing agent which promotes healthy granulation and stimulates epithelial proliferation. It is indicated for obstinate ulceration where the peripheral circulation is good. It is apt to be irritant and is contra-indicated for fresh wounds or where the peripheral circulation is poor. It is generally used as Scarlet Red Ointment, a smear of ointment being applied to the edge of the ulcer only. A soothing ointment may be used for alternate treatments with the Scarlet Red Ointment. The stains of scarlet red may be removed with benzene.

Scarlet Red Ointment (*Unguentum Rubrum Scarlatinum*) B.P.C. 1954 is 5 per cent of Scarlet Red in Simple Ointment to 100 per cent.

SILICONES

Silicones are polymers with structures consisting of alternate atoms of silicon and oxygen, organic groups such as methyl- or phenyl-being attached to the silicon atoms.

Silicones are water-repellent and have a low surface tension. Silicones may be used as barrier creams for protecting the skin against water-soluble irritants and also as lubricants and inert vehicles for emulsions and aerosols.

Dimethicone B.P.C. syn. Dimethyl Silicone fluid has the general formula of $CH_3(Si[CH_3]_2O)_n \cdot Si(CH_3)_3$

The B.P.C. describes five dimethicones of varying molecular weights all of which are clear colourless liquids. Silicone must make up 20 per cent of the preparation before it is effective.

Proprietary brands:

"Atrixo Hand Care" (Smith & Nephew) is an oil-in-water emulsion containing silicone in a vanishing cream base and is used to prevent dryness of the skin especially where the skin is frequently immersed in water.

"Dispray Silicone" (Pigot & Smith) is a pressurized spray containing Castor Oil 3·5 per cent, Terpineol 0·35 per cent in Silicone Fluid and Industrial Methylated Spirit with a propellant and is used in the prevention and treatment of bedsores.

"Rikospray Silicone" (Riker) is an aerosol using silicone as a vehicle with active constituents of aluminium dihydroxyallantoinate and cetyl pyridinium chloride and is also used in the treatment of bedsores.

"Conotrane" (Ward, Blenkinsop) is a cream containing 20 per cent Dimethicone and 0·05 per cent of Hydrargaphen.

"Siopel Cream" (ICI Pharmaceuticals) contains 0·3 per cent of Cetrimide in an oil-in-water cream containing silicone fluid and is used to prevent bedsores and in the treatment of occupational dermatoses.

"Siopel Spray" (ICI Pharmaceuticals) is a pressurized spray pack containing a silicone fluid dissolved in surgical spirit and is used in the treatment of bedsores.

SILVER NITRATE

Silver Nitrate (*Argenti Nitras*) B.P. occurs as colourless tabular crystals with a bitter metallic taste, containing not less than 99·8 per cent of $AgNO_3$.

Silver nitrate and preparations of silver nitrate should be stored away from light, in glass-stoppered bottles of coloured glass. Silver nitrate is soluble 2 parts in 1 part of water, and 1 in 27 of 95 per cent Alcohol.

Silver nitrate is incompatible with organic materials, tartaric acid, alkalies and acids and salts of halogen acids, such as ferric chloride.

Antidote. The immediate application of a compress of a 10 per cent aqueous solution of sodium chloride, or a foot-bath of strong saline solution will relieve pain due to silver nitrate. Silver chloride is formed.

Recent stains of silver nitrate may be removed from the skin by the application of potassium iodide to the moistened stain and leaving for a few hours. To remove recent stains from cloth, apply a 10 per cent solution of potassium iodide and remove the yellow stain produced with a 10 per cent solution of sodium thiosulphate.

Care should be taken when applying silver nitrate to patients having fair, dry skins because these are more likely to react severely to silver nitrate. On the other hand, for patients having very moist, hyperidrotic skins a stronger solution than usual may be required. The skin will be saturated with sodium chloride from the sweat, and the sodium chloride will react with the silver nitrate to form silver chloride.

Toughened Silver Nitrate (Argenti Nitras Induratus) B.P. is prepared by fusing 95 per cent of Silver Nitrate with 5 per cent of Potassium Nitrate and moulding the product into suitable shapes. Toughened Silver Nitrate should be stored away from the light. Special holders for Toughened Silver Nitrate are available and are very convenient. Sticks of Toughened Silver Nitrate may be stored in Burnt Alum.

Silver Nitrate, Mitigated (Argenti Nitras Mitigatus) B.P.C. contains 33 per cent of silver nitrate moulded into sticks with potassium nitrate. In ordering a "Silver Nitrate Stick" it should be remembered that, ordinarily, Silver Nitrate, Mitigated, will be supplied unless Toughened Silver Nitrate is specified.

Silver nitrate is antiseptic, astringent (below 20 per cent), irritant and caustic (above 25 per cent). As with salicylic acid, silver nitrate is rarely used as an antiseptic *per se*; its antiseptic properties are incidental to the other uses to which it is put.

It is for its astringent and caustic properties that silver nitrate is chiefly used in chiropody. Although it has been suggested that silver nitrate is astringent below 20 per cent strength and caustic above 25 per cent this is an arbitrary division. It is not possible to define explicitly where astringent action ends and caustic action begins.

When applied to the skin, it is said that silver nitrate combines with the skin proteins to form a thick layer of silver albuminate, which at first is white, but gradually changes to brown and, later, to black under the influence of light. Because it forms an insoluble barrier by combining with the tissue chlorides, silver nitrate does not penetrate very deeply. It would seem that the action of silver nitrate on the skin takes place very rapidly. Even if it is neutralized with sodium chloride immediately after it has been applied, a black coagulum will still be formed. The degree of silver nitrate action does not depend solely on the strength of the solution which is applied. The amount of solution used and the way in which it is applied influence the action to a very marked degree. If a 20 per cent solution of silver nitrate is painted on to, say, a soft corn, its action will be very superficial; but if the 20 per cent solution is rubbed into the soft corn it will produce a much stronger reaction and will penetrate much more deeply. Silver nitrate is a drug which works most effectively if applied at frequent intervals. It has already been noted that it is apparently effective very rapidly and there seems, therefore, to be very little advantage in leaving silver nitrate on for long periods between treatments. It is well worth spending some time in finding out the effect of rubbing silver nitrate into lesions instead of using it as paint. Not only will it be found to be a much more useful medicament than is generally realized, but also the more dilute solutions can be used, an important point in view of the fact that it may also be used for many of the purposes listed for the 25 and 50 per cent solutions if it is rubbed into the lesion concerned.

20–25 per cent may be used in the treatment of soft corns. The solution is generally applied at fortnightly intervals, the coagulum being completely removed before further solution is applied. A shorter interval than 14 days between treatments is to be preferred if this is possible. The 25 per cent solution serves as a useful foil to 25 per cent ointment of salicylic acid and may be used with it alternately. The 25 per cent solution may also be applied to a relaxed nail sulcus, but in this case better results are achieved if the solution is merely painted on. The solution may be applied to hard corns and to areas of callus, particularly if the callus is macerated.

40–50 per cent may be applied to vascular corns or deep hard corns at weekly or fortnightly intervals and to excess granulation tissue every 3 or 4 days. This strength may occasionally be applied to warts. In every case the coagulum from the previous treatment must be removed before fresh solution is applied.

Toughened Silver Nitrate. Before the Toughened Silver Nitrate stick is applied it is moistened with water. It should not be moistened with spirit, because the strongest solution which can be produced in spirit is about 4 per cent. The silver nitrate stick must never be moistened in the instrument tray. This practice will rapidly cause damage to instruments.

Because of the solubility of silver nitrate in water, the toughened silver nitrate stick will form a 200 per cent solution when rubbed into the skin in the presence of an excess amount of water, or a lower strength solution depending on the quantity of water present. For surgery use, it may be that the saturated (200 per cent)[1] solution is a better way of keeping such a corrosive medicament safely. A small coloured glass bottle with a plastic screw top may be used to keep this strength solution which may then be applied to the skin by means of a wooden applicator stick. For the solution to be saturated there must be undissolved crystals at the bottom of the bottle.

Toughened Silver Nitrate or 200 per cent solution may be applied to vascular corns, especially on the plantar surface. The return period is about 14 days, although silver nitrate may safely be left on for longer periods. This strength may be applied to excessive granulation tissue when this occurs as a complication to onychocryptosis. In this case the return period should be 3–7 days. The use of 200 per cent in the treatment of warts should be regarded as an auxiliary to other forms of treatment, the stick may be used alone to clear up the final fragments of a wart. Silver nitrate, when used alone, should not be given for more than two consecutive occasions, otherwise the treatment of the wart may be prolonged. Silver nitrate assists in the diagnosis of a doubtful wart. If the suspected lesion is rubbed with Toughened Silver Nitrate or with a 10 per cent solution of silver nitrate and is then exposed to a bright light or to the infra-red lamp, the characteristic mosaic pattern should appear in from 5–10 minutes.

Methargen is Silver 2, 2'-methylene*bis* (Naphthalene-3-sulphonate). It is an antiseptic applied topically as a 1 per cent solution, a 1 per cent water miscible cream, a 1 per cent oil-in-water emulsion or as a tulle.

Methargen is for use on burns, varicose ulcers and superficial lesions. It is useful in the treatment of septic conditions. Contact with metal causes a chemical reaction to take place and a metal spatula introduced into a jar of this medicament is enough to cause the whole amount to become discoloured and useless.

"Methargen Gauze (Tulle) Dressings" are cotton or rayon tulle impregnated with a soft water-soluble basis consisting of a mixture of macrogols and Methargen 1 per cent.

"Viacutan" (Ward, Blenkinsop) is Methargen available as a coloured 1 per cent solution, water miscible cream, an oil-in-water emulsion or as a tulle.

SOAP (see also Detergents, page 33)

Soft Soap (*Sapo Mollis*) B.P. is a yellowish-white to green, or brown unctuous substance obtained by the interaction of sodium or

[1] See page 4.

potassium hydroxide with suitable vegetable oils or with fatty acids. It is soluble in water and alcohol.

Crude soft soap which contains some residual potassium hydroxide may be used in the treatment of hard and extensive callus. The foot is first soaked in water and the crude soft soap is then rubbed into the wet callus. This operation may be carried out with the foot still in the water. The soft soap is left on for about a quarter of an hour and the foot is then immersed again in warm water. The hard callus should be softened by the action of the free potassium hydroxide. This method of treatment may be compared with the treatment of warts using potassium hydroxide, the principles involved are exactly the same. The crude soft soap may be thought of as an ointment of potassium hydroxide. Alternatively, after the crude soft soap has been applied to the callus, it may be covered with lint and bandage and left in position for a week. It will be noted that the use of soft soap to soften callus is inconvenient in many ways, and it is therefore reserved for cases which cannot be dealt with by other methods. A solution of soft soap in I.M.S. may be used to cleanse the skin.

Soft soap is also useful during the manufacture of appliances as a parting-agent to prevent plaster of paris sticking to casts or to the skin.

SODIUM SALTS

Sodium Bicarbonate (*Sodii Bicarbonas*) B.P. occurs as a white powder or small crystals containing not less than 99·0 per cent of $NaHCO_3$. It is soluble 1 part in 11 parts of water.

Sodium bicarbonate may be used in the preparation of carbon dioxide foot-baths (see Carbon Dioxide) and should also be on hand for use as a neutralizing agent in the event of an accident with an acid.

Sodium Chloride (*Sodii Chloridum*) B.P. syn. Common Salt occurs as colourless crystals or as a white powder containing not less than 99·5 per cent of NaCl. It is soluble 1 part in 3 parts of water, 1 in 10 of glycerin and 1 in 200 of alcohol.

Solutions of salt inhibit the multiplication of bacteria by osmotic action and, what is probably more important, they stimulate the flow of lymph.

Normal Saline Solution is a 0·9 per cent aqueous solution of sodium chloride. It is isotonic with the liquid of the blood corpuscles and exerts the same osmotic pressure as the blood fluid. Normal saline solution is used for cleaning out cavities, for dressing septic wounds and as a vehicle for drugs such as the acridines.

Saline foot-baths are useful, administered at home by the patient, for the treatment of septic conditions and for breakdowns caused by the action of acids during the treatment of warts. A dessertspoonful of salt should be added to every pint of water used or 12 ml. to 1 litre. If the treatment of warts with acids has caused pain, the patient should be instructed to immerse the foot in a warm saline foot-bath, without removing the dressing.

Sodium Polymetaphosphate B.P.C. syn. Sodium Hexametaphosphate is colourless plates or powder containing not less than 85 per cent of $(NaPO_3)_x$ and 8–15 per cent of $Na_4P_2O_7$. It dissolves slowly in water and is insoluble in organic solvents.

Sodium polymetaphosphate may be used as a 5 per cent dusting-powder in bromidrosis and hyperidrosis, and as a prophylactic against fungal infection of the feet. Sodium polymetaphosphate may be added to the water in which instruments are boiled to prevent corrosion. It is used in domestic water softeners.

"Calgon" (Albright and Wilson) is a brand of sodium polymetaphosphate.

Sodium Fusidate (see Antibiotics)

Sodium Lauryl Sulphate (*Sodii et Laurylis Sulphas*) B.P. is a mixture of sodium normal primary alkyl sulphates, consisting chiefly of sodium dodecyl sulphate and containing the equivalent of not less than 58 per cent w/w of total alcohols. It occurs as white or pale yellow crystals or powder and is readily soluble in water. It is incompatible with cationic materials such as chlorhexidine and with strong acids.

Sodium lauryl sulphate is a detergent and wetting agent and will reduce surface tension. It is bacteriostatic for Gram-positive bacteria but is ineffective against many Gram-negative organisms. It is used in the preparation of double phase water-miscible semi-solids, being an anionic emulgent and, mixed with 90 per cent cetostearyl alcohol, is used to make emulsifying wax.

"Teepol 610" (Shell Chemicals) is an aqueous solution of sodium secondary alkyl sulphates. This anionic detergent may be used for general cleansing of glassware, metal and plastic surfaces, etc., as a 1 per cent aqueous solution. Teepol may also be used as an anti-mist solution for spectacles or lenses, being applied in solution form and then rubbed bright.

There are many other proprietary preparations of Alkyl Sulphates including: "Comprox" (B.P.—Evans Chemicals), "Cycloryl" (Cyclo Chemicals), "Empicol" (Marchon), "Ethisan" (Ethica Laboratories), "Pentrone" (Glovers), "ProDermide" (Kerfoot), "Sipon E.S." (Sipon) and "Sulphonated Lorol" (Ronsheim & Moore).

STARCH

Starch (*Amylum*) B.P. is a fine white powder which may be obtained from maize (*Zea mays*), rice (*Oryza sativa*), wheat (*Triticum aestivum*) and potato (*Solanum tuberosum*). It is incompatible with iodine.

Starch should be stored in a well-closed container in a cool, dry place. It is absorbent and soothing and is widely used in dusting-powders. It absorbs its own weight of moisture, but has a tendency to cake.

Starch Glycerin (*Glycerinum Amyli*) B.P.C. 1963 is 8·5 per cent of Wheat Starch heated with 17 per cent of water and 74·5 per cent of Glycerin to a temperature not over 140° F. until the mixture gelatinizes. This preparation does not store well and should be freshly prepared.

Starch Glycerin may be used for chilblains and is specific for the treatment of iodine rash and iodine burns. It may also be employed in the treatment of plaster dermatitis. It is applied spread thinly on lint.

Starch is an ingredient of Compound Zinc Paste B.P. and Zinc and Salicylic Acid Paste B.P. (see under Zinc).

Starch is used as a lubricant in *Absorbable Dusting Powder* B.P. which is prepared from Maize Starch containing not more than 2 per cent of magnesium oxide which is included to keep it in the form of a free flowing powder and to increase its lubricating properties. In particular it is used for lubricating surgeon's gloves.

Starch is also a basic ingredient of many dusting-powders including:

Chlorphenesin Dusting-powder B.P.C.

Talc Dusting-powder B.P.C.

Zinc and Salicylic Acid Dusting-powder B.P.C.

Zinc, Starch and Talc Dusting-powder B.P.C.

Zinc Undecenoate Dusting-powder B.P.C.

N.B.: Note that "Dusting Powder" is not hyphenated in the official title "Absorbable Dusting Powder".

TALC

Purified Talc (*Talcum Purificatum*) B.P.C. syn. French Chalk is a native hydrated magnesium silicate, $Mg_6(Si_2O_5)_4(OH)_4$. It is a grey amorphous powder, which is completely insoluble in water and acids.

Talc is used as a lubricant in massage powders up to 100 per cent and in dusting-powders up to 50 per cent as an absorbent and antipruritic.

Talc is less absorbent than kaolin or starch. Being of natural

origin, talc is subject to bacterial contamination and should have
been carefully sterilized before being dispensed; nevertheless it is a
wise precaution not to apply talc to any open wound or abrasion.

Talc is an ingredient of:

Chlorphenesin Dusting-powder B.P.C.

Talc Dusting-powder B.P.C. contains 90 per cent Talc, 10 per cent
Starch.

Zinc, Starch and Talc Dusting-powder B.P.C.

TANNIC ACID

Tannic acid was formerly much used as an astringent, particularly
on burns. Its use has now been virtually discontinued.

Borotannic Complex is an ester of borotrioxybenzoic acid and is
used as an anti-mycotic paint on nails and on skin. It is said to act
by producing an acid environment and by its drying and astringent
action, both of which are unfavourable to mycotic growth.

"Medistan" (Lloyds' Pharmaceuticals) is a paint containing Borotannic Complex 9·92 per cent in Ethyl Acetate and Alcohol.

"Phytex" (Wynlit Laboratories) is a paint containing Borotannic
Complex 9 per cent with Salicylic Acid 1 per cent in Ethyl Acetate
and Alcohol. This replaces "Onycho Phytex" and "Dermato Phytex".

TARTARIC ACID (see Acetic Acid)

TERPINEOL

Terpineol (*Terpineol*) B.P., $C_{10}H_{17}OH$, is a mixture of isomers
obtained by fractionation from terpin hydrate. It is a colourless,
slightly viscous liquid which is very slightly soluble in water, and is
soluble 1 part in 2 parts of alcohol (70 per cent).

Terpineol has antiseptic properties and is used as a solvent in
Solution of Chloroxylenol and in similar proprietary preparations
(see Halogenated Phenols—Chloroxylenol).

THIOMERSAL (see Mercury)

TRICHLOROACETIC ACID

Trichloroacetic Acid (*Acidum Trichloraceticum*) B.P. syn. Tri-
chloracetic Acid occurs as very deliquescent crystals containing not
less than 98·0 per cent of $CCl_3 \cdot COOH$. Trichloroacetic acid should
be stored in moisture-excluding containers. The crystals are readily
soluble in water, alcohol and ether.

Trichloroacetic acid is caustic, keratolytic and astringent and is used in the treatment of warts. Although it is chemically a stronger acid than monochloroacetic acid, it is generally considered that its action is less drastic and more superficial than that of the latter. This is true if the acid is merely painted on to a lesion; if a crystal or the saturated solution of trichloroacetic acid is rubbed well into a wart, an extensive breakdown may be caused. The combination of trichloroacetic acid with salicylic acid will be found to be much more drastic than the combination of monochloroacetic acid and salicylic acid. It is probably safe to say that the action of trichloroacetic acid is more easily *controlled* than that of monochloroacetic acid or of salicylic acid and it is for this reason that it may be used as in method 1 (*a*) below when there is little adipose tissue between wart and underlying periosteum, e.g. warts occurring over joints. Trichloroacetic acid is apt to harden warts which may then, if necessary, be softened with Potassium Hydroxide Solution.

Techniques of Application

1 (*a*). After removing the superficial layers of the wart, the growth is soaked with saturated solution of trichloroacetic acid. The return period should be not less than 4 days.

1 (*b*). After removing the superficial layers, a crystal of the acid is gently rubbed into the growth for a timed period. (Use 30 seconds as a starting dose.) This produces a much stronger reaction than method 1 (*a*). The return period is from 4–14 days.

2. After removing the superficial layers, the growth is first soaked with the saturated solution and then rubbed with moistened Toughened Silver Nitrate. This is repeated until there are several layers of trichloroacetic acid and silver nitrate the final layer being of silver nitrate. The foot may be immersed in water after the first twenty-four hours. The minimum return period is 4 days. When the patient returns, there will be a tough black coagulum which frequently tends to curl up at the edges and which may sometimes be peeled off with forceps after the foot has been immersed in a warm foot-bath. This method is particularly suitable for large shallow growths of the "mosaic" variety as well as for small "daughter" growths and also for growths occurring in the nail groove or interdigitally.

3. Trichloroacetic acid may be used in conjunction with salicylic acid by methods similar to No. II given for salicylic acid described on page 193. It must be remembered that trichloroacetic acid will give a much stronger reaction than monochloroacetic acid if this technique is used.

UNDECENOIC ACID

Undecenoic Acid (*Acidum Undecenoicum*) B.P. syn. Undecylinic Acid, is a long-chain fatty acid with a formula:

$$CH_2{:}CH{\cdot}(CH_2)_8{\cdot}COOH$$

It occurs as a yellow liquid, or yellow crystalline masses, and has a characteristic odour. Undecenoic acid is almost insoluble in water but is miscible with alcohol and ether.

The use of undecenoic acid and its zinc salts is becoming increasingly popular for the treatment of superficial mycotic infections. It is effective against the gypseum group of *Trichophyton, T. purpureum, Epidermophyton floccosum, Microsporum audouini* and *Candida albicans*. It is most effective in a vanishing cream base or it may be used in powder form in concentrations of 2–15 per cent.

Zinc Undecenoate Dusting-powder B.P.C. contains Undecenoic Acid 2 per cent, Zinc Undecenoate 10 per cent, Starch 50 per cent, Pumilo Pine Oil 0·5 per cent and Light Kaolin to 100 per cent.

Zinc Undecenoate Ointment B.P. contains 5 per cent of Undecenoic Acid, 20 per cent of Zinc Undecenoate in Emulsifying Ointment.

"Mycota Cream" (Boots) contains Undecenoic Acid 5 per cent, Zinc Undecenoate 20 per cent in a water-miscible basis.

"Mycota Powder" (Boots) contains Undecenoic Acid 2 per cent and Zinc Undecenoate 20 per cent.

"Tineafax Ointment" (Burroughs Wellcome) contains 8 per cent of Zinc Undecenoate with zinc naphthenate, mesulphen, Methyl Salicylate, Terpineol and Chlorocresol.

"Tineafax Powder" (Burroughs Wellcome) contains 10 per cent Zinc Undecenoate.

"Amoxal" (Smith & Nephew) Dusting-powder contains 2 per cent Pentalamide, 0·5 per cent Hexachlorophane.

"Episol" (Crookes) Dusting-powder contains 0·5 per cent Halethazole.

"Phytocil" (Wade) Dusting-powder contains 5·8 per cent Zinc Undecylenate.

WOOL ALCOHOLS (see Fats, Animal)

WOOL FAT (see Fats, Animal)

ZINC SALTS

Salts of Zinc are incompatible with alkalies, alkaline carbonates and with vegetable infusions.

Zinc Oxide (*Zinci Oxidum*) B.P. is a fine, white, amorphous powder containing not less than 99·0 per cent of ZnO. It is insoluble in water and alcohol, but is soluble in dilute acids and in ammonia.

Zinc oxide tends to absorb moisture from the air and should be stored in air-tight containers. It is sometimes loosely referred to as "Zinc". Zinc oxide is a mild astringent and antiseptic and is used in soothing and protective applications. It will absorb about one and a half times its own weight of moisture. It is an ingredient of a large number of official preparations many of which have been discussed above.

Calamine Application Compound B.P.C. and *Calamine Cream, Aqueous* see Calamine B.P.C.

Zinc Cream (*Cremor Zinci Oxidi*) B.P. contains 32 per cent of Zinc Oxide in a cream basis.

Zinc and Ichthammol Cream B.P.C. see Ichthammol.

Chlorphenesin Dusting-powder B.P.C. see Chlorphenesin.

Zinc and Salicylic Acid Dusting-powder B.P.C. see Salicylic Acid.

Zinc, Starch and Talc Dusting-powder B.P.C. contains 25 per cent of Zinc Oxide, 25 per cent of Starch, 50 per cent of Talc.

Zinc Gelatin B.P.C. syn. Unna's Paste contains 15 per cent of Zinc Oxide, 15 per cent of Gelatin, 35 per cent of Glycerin in water to 100 per cent.

Calamine Lotion B.P. see Calamine.

Benzocaine Ointment, Compound B.P.C. see Benzocaine.

Zinc Ointment (*Unguentum Zinci Oxidi*) B.P. contains 15 per cent of Zinc Oxide in Simple Ointment.

Zinc Paste, Compound B.P. contains 25 per cent of Zinc Oxide, 25 per cent of Starch in White Soft Paraffin.

Zinc and Salicylic Acid Paste (*Pasta Zinci Oxidi cum Acido Salicylico*) B.P. syn. Lassar's Paste see Salicylic Acid.

Zinc Stearate (*Zinci Stearas*) B.P.C. is a white amorphous powder consisting chiefly of Zinc Stearate, $Zn(C_{18}H_{35}O_2)_2$ with variable quantities of zinc oleate and zinc palminate.

Zinc stearate is a soothing and astringent powder used in dusting-powders. It is indicated in plaster dermatitis, hyperidrosis and bromidrosis. A powder consisting of 95 parts of Zinc Stearate and 5 parts of Flowers of Sulphur is useful for treating hyperidrosis. Calamine Application, Compound B.P.C. contains 2·5 per cent of Zinc Stearate.

Zinc Sulphate (*Zinci Sulphas*) B.P. occurs as a crystalline powder, or colourless crystals and contains not less than 99·5 per cent of $ZnSO_4, 7H_2O$. Zinc stearate is very soluble in water but insoluble in alcohol.

Zinc sulphate is astringent, antiseptic, mildly caustic and irritant. Zinc Sulphate Lotion may be used to stimulate ulcers which are slow to heal. Copper and Zinc Sulphates Lotion is astringent and antiseptic.

Copper and Zinc Sulphates Lotion (Lotio Cupri et Zinci Sulphatum) B.P.C. syn. Dalibour Water contains 1·5 per cent Zinc Sulphate, 1 per cent Copper Sulphate in Camphor Water.

Zinc Sulphate Lotion (Lotio Zinci Sulphatis) B.P.C. syn. Lotio Rubra contains 1 per cent Zinc Sulphate, 1 per cent Amaranth Solution in water. (N.B. Red Lotion has nothing to do with Scarlet Red.)

Zinc Undecenoate (*Zinci Undecenoas*) B.P. occurs as a fine white or creamy-white powder which is almost insoluble in water and alcohol.

Zinc Undecenoate is a fungicide which is becoming increasingly popular in the treatment of dermatophytosis (see Undecenoic Acid, page 219).

INDEX

See also Addenda p. 238

Latin names have been omitted from the index. Preparations such as Ointments are listed under the drug from which they take their title and alphabetical reference lists appear under the title Ointment, Paste, etc. There are cross-references liking conditions to drugs and, in some cases, drugs to conditions.

223

Hydrogen-ion concentration, 8
Hydrogen Peroxide Solution, 29, **180**
nail debris, 126; sepsis, 81
Hydrostatic pressure, 46
Hydrous Ointment, see Oily Cream
Hydrous Wool Fat, 173
Hydrous Wool Fat Ointment, 173
Hydroxysuccinic Acid, syn.: Malic
Acid
Hyperidrosis, 110
Alum, 144; Aluminium Acetate, 144;
Chloroxyienol, 177; Formalin,
174; Menthol, 190; Potassium
Hydroxyquinoline Sulphate, 202;
Potassium Permanganate, 202;
Salicylic Acid, 205; Sodium Poly-
metaphosphate, 215; Zinc
Stearate, 234
Hyperkeratosis, 99, 122
See also callus
Hypertonic solutions, 8
"Hyposan", see Chlorinated Lime, 164

"Ibcol", see Chloroxylenol, 177
Ichthammol, 37, **181**
chilblains, 95, 96; fissures, 118;
plaster dermatitis, 124; sepsis, 84;
ulceration, 108
Ichthammol and Zinc Cream, 181
Ichthammol Glycerin, 181
Ichthammol in Collodion, 181, 210
Ichthammol Ointment, 181
Ichthosulphol, syn.: Ichthammol
Ichthyol, syn.: Ichthammol
"Id", "Ide"—conditions, 121
Immunity, 60
I.M.S., syn.: Industrial Methylated
Spirit
Incandescent Light Bulbs, 21
Incompatibility, 137
Industrial Methylated Spirit, 8, **141**
See also Alcohol
Infected wounds, see sepsis
Infected wounds, repair of, 56
Infection, airborne, 76; focal, 64;
spread of, 65; tissue response to,
61; prevention of, see antisepsis,
asepsis, instrument sterilization;
treatment of, see sepsis
Inflammation, **40–60**
degrees of, 57; treatment of (aseptic),
89; treatment of (septic), 80
Infra-red radiations, 21, 82, 92
Instrument sterilization, 74
Alcohol, 142; Benzalkonium Chlor-
ide, 150; Cetrimide, 162; Chlor-

hexidine, 177; Chloroxylenol, 177;
Cresol, 160; Phenol, 198; Sodium
Polymetaphosphate, 222
Interface, 5
Intertrigo, 121
"Intralgin", see Benzocaine, 151
"Iodex", see Iodine, 184
Iodine, 1, 28, 38, **182**
blisters, 116; bursitis, 92, 93; chil-
blains, 94; callus and corns, 100,
102; fungal infections, 120, 122;
onychomycosis, 122; post-opera-
tive, 77; pre-operative, 71; syno-
vitis, 92
Iodine burns, 182
Sodium Thiosulphate, 182; Starch,
216
Iodine Ointment, Non-staining, 183
Iodine Ointment, Non-staining with
Methyl Salicylate, 183
Iodine rash, 182
Iodine Solution Aqueous, 183
Iodine Solution Strong, 183
Iodine Solution Weak, 183
"Iodobenz", 184
Iodochlorhydroxyquinoline, 184
Iodophores, 184
Ionization, 34
Iron salts, 184
Isopropanol, syn.: Isopropyl Alcohol
Isopropyl Alcohol, 1, 8, 77, **142**
See also Alcohol
Isotonic solution, 7

"Jadit", see Buclosamide, 165
"Jelonet", see Paraffin Gauze Dressing,
131
"Jeypine", see Chloroxylenol, 177
"Jeysol", see Cresol, 163
"Johnson's First Aid Cream", see
Dibromopropamidine, 170

Kaolin, 12, 13, 15, **185**
bursitis, 92; callus, 101; chilblains,
95; sepsis, 81, 83
Kaolin Poultice, 185
Kelly's Paint, see Pyroxylin, 204
Keratinization, 97
Keratolytics, **31, 32**
"Kling" Bandage, see Conforming
Bandage, 128
"Kymol", see Cresol, 168

Lactic Acid, 186
warts, 107
"Lacto-calamine", see Calamine, 156

ADDENDA